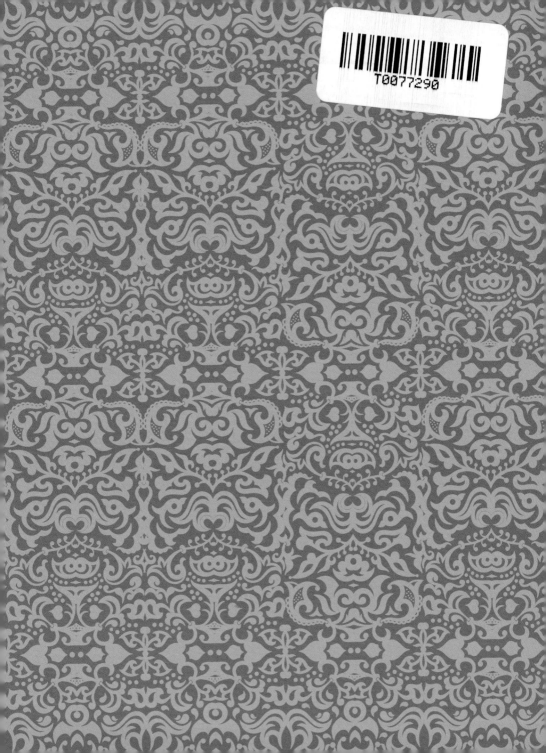

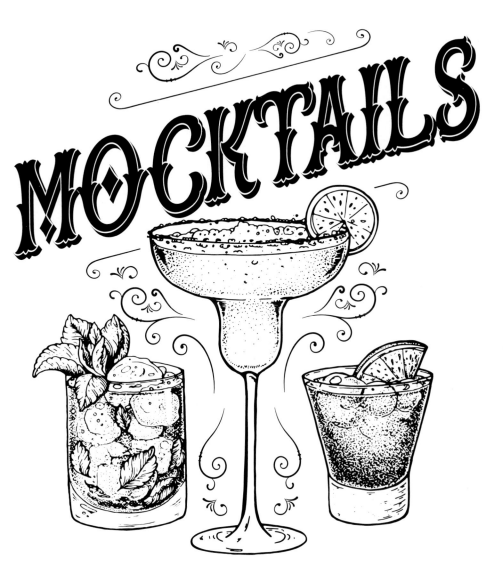

MOCKTAILS

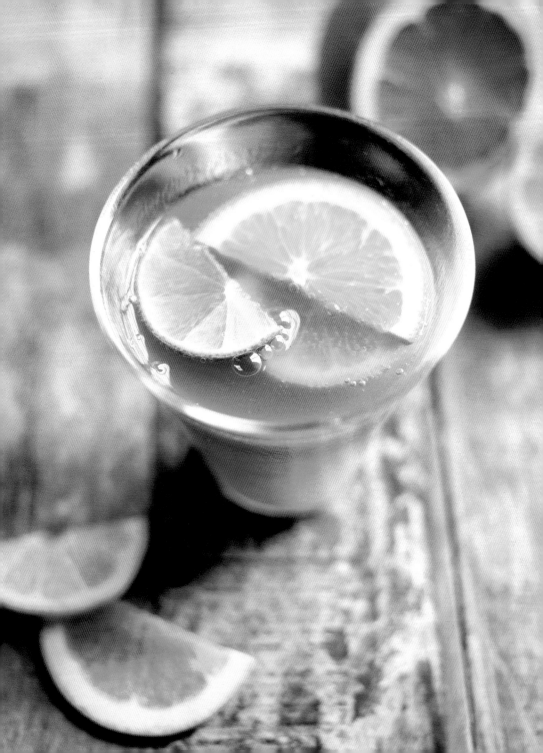

THE ART OF MIXOLOGY™

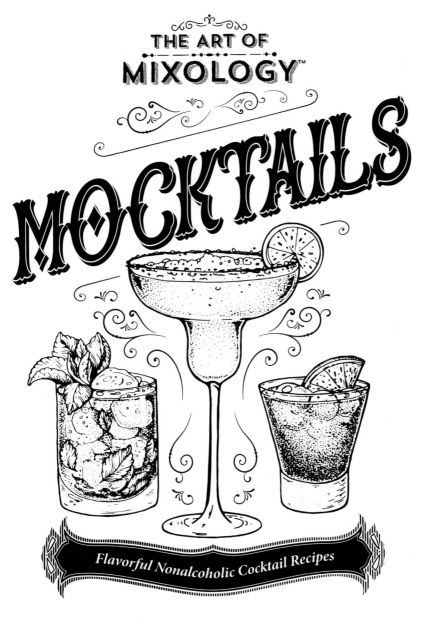

MOCKTAILS

Flavorful Nonalcoholic Cocktail Recipes

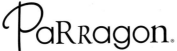

PaRragon®

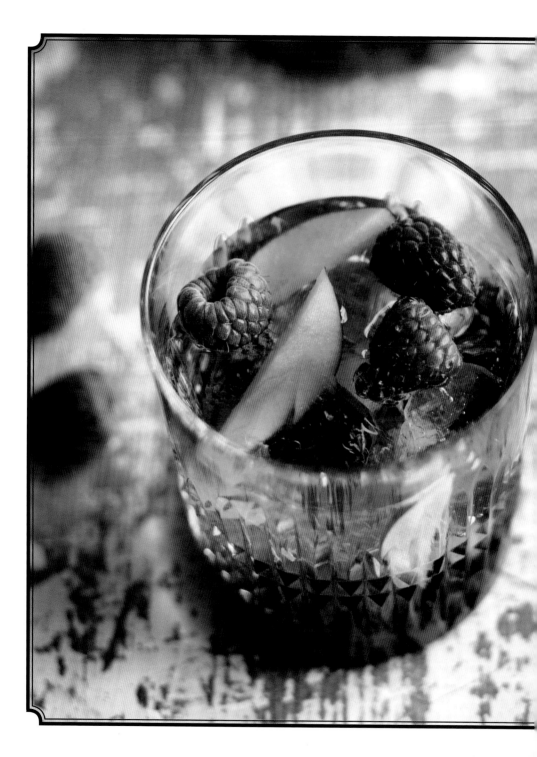

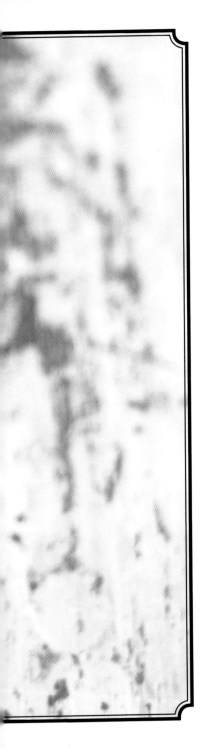

CONTENTS

THE RISE OF THE MOCKTAIL

The word "mocktail" is a marriage of "mock" and "cocktail." While there is no recorded date for when these nonalcoholic drinks first became popular, the word itself was coined in 1979 in an advertisement for a glassware brand. The concept of mocktails must, however, predate this. As long as people have drunk in bars, bartenders will have needed to provide tempting libations for any customers who wished to steer clear of the hard stuff.

Nonalcoholic beverages became more popular during the Prohibition years in the United States (1920–1933). This led to the creation of the soda jerk, a person who operated soda fountains in drugstores throughout the United States. The soda jerk would create drinks in tall glasses, using flavored syrups mixed with carbonated water and topped with one or two scoops of ice cream. These were served with a long-handled spoon and drinking straws—this trend reached its height in the 1940s.

While outlawing alcohol during Prohibition negatively affected the previously burgeoning cocktail culture, it also created a renaissance for temperance drinks. These concoctions could be time-consuming to make and surprisingly complex. As a result, people started to experiment with more interesting ingredients including shrubs, syrups, and fresh fruit, a trend that we are seeing again in the creation of modern-day cocktails and mocktails.

Today, the mocktail revolution is just behind the cocktail revival. Bartenders are spending as much time creating mocktails with complex flavor profiles as they spend creating cocktails. There is a large market for quality mocktails and this is likely to be driven by

a mainstream interest in living a healthy lifestyle and cutting out processed ingredients and excess sugar from our diet. Good-quality nonalcoholic offerings also appeal to a broad range of people—from pregnant women to athletes and many in between—so it is worth planning the creation of your mocktails in the same way as you would your alcoholic drinks.

This book will give you ideas for making mocktails at home or in the bar, and can also be used as a guide for experimenting. Just remember that the process of making drinks can be as much fun as drinking them!

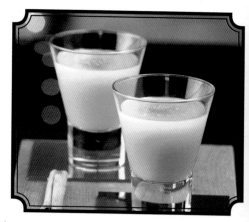

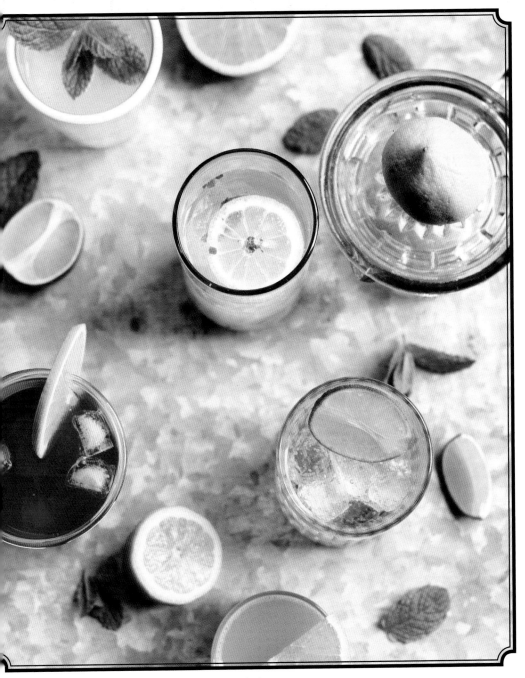

INGREDIENTS

Any mixed drink relies on an appropriate combination of ingredients to endow it with mixology magic. There is a wide variety of ingredients suitable for mocktails—shown below are the main categories that you will encounter in this book, and that you can use as you start to experiment with your own mocktails.

Juices

Juices come in a number of forms, ranging from freshly squeezed juices and store-bought brands to pulps and fruit nectars. Whichever you choose for your mocktails, remember that freshly squeezed juice will give you the purest tasting experience and the best-quality drinks. You can make your own juices at home using an electric juicer, a hand juicer, or even just by giving the fruit sections a good squeeze by hand. Freshly squeezed juice will need to be strained to remove any bits.

Syrups

Syrups, a combination of sugar and water, are used all over the world by mixologists, baristas, and chefs both to sweeten and add flavor to their creations. There is a huge variety of brands that create flavored syrups such as cola, vanilla, bubble gum, and rosemary, but it is also easy to create your own. Some of the mocktail recipes here tell you how to make your own syrups; others use store-bought syrups. There is also a practical guide to making your own syrup on page 113.

Shrubs

A shrub is a slightly acidic liquid traditionally made with fruit, sugar, and vinegar. The name "shrub" is derived from an Arabic word meaning "to drink." The idea of shrubs originates from the creation of medicinal cordials in the 15th century. Shrubs were also popular in colonial America, then mixed with cool water to provide a pick-me-up on hot days, as well as during the Prohibition era, providing a tasty, thirst-quenching beverage with no alcohol.

A proper shrub has a flavor that is both sweet and tart, so it stimulates the appetite while also enching thirst. Shrubs are easy to make home, and for mocktail lovers they're o quite versatile. If you are prepared for a nmer of shrub-making, you can start with awberries when they come into season, d move through the berries and fruits as ey mature over the summer. Some of the ocktail recipes here tell you how to make ur own shrubs. There is also a practical ide to making your own shrub on page 149.

a and Coffee

a has been used for centuries as a delicious verage, both hot and cold. With a huge riety of teas including bagged, loose-leaf, rbal, and even matcha powder, there is a ver-ending list of possible flavors. There are any uses for tea within mocktails, including fusions, chilled tea, and tea syrups.

offee has grown in popularity as an ingredient mixed drinks over the past few years. There e many ways to use coffee in mocktails, nging from using the beans as a garnish or ing iced coffee as an ingredient to create ffee-flavored syrups. When creating your n flavors you can use both the bean and ound coffee depending on the style and vor profile you are aiming to achieve.

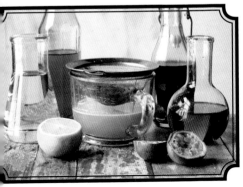

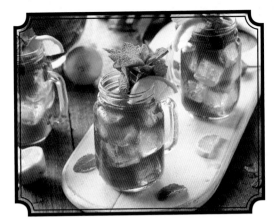

Purees

A puree is an easy way to enhance a mocktail with fruity flavors without needing to muddle fruit directly into your mixed drink. To make your own puree at home, prepare your fruit and place it in a blender or food processor with sugar and lemon juice and process for around 30 seconds. Pour into a fine sieve set over a bowl, press the liquid through the sieve with a rubber spatula, and discard the solids. You can make a puree using any fruit or vegetable with a high juice content.

Herbs and Spices

When bartenders get creative and design new mixed drinks, many techniques and ingredients are borrowed from the kitchen. One of these includes the use of herbs and spices. Ingredients such as cinnamon, basil, cardamom, and lavender have found their way into the bartender's repertoire to create delicious mocktails. There are also many classic, internationally recognized drinks that use fresh mint. There are many ways to use these fresh, fragrant ingredients such as in infusions, syrups, and shrubs.

GLASSWARE

How you present and serve your drinks is crucial in any form of mixology. You need to serve a mocktail in the appropriate glass—the size, shape and style all have an impact on the perception and enjoyment of the drink. Here are some of the classic glasses that you will likely have in your collection, although be aware that there are no set rules.

Martini Glass

The most iconic of all mixed drink glasses, the conical martini glass emerged with the Art Deco movement. The glass has a low, wide bowl and the long stem is perfect for chilled drinks as it keeps people's hands from inadvertently warming the cocktail.

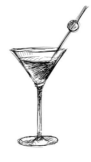

Highball Glass

Sometimes also known as a Collins glass, these glasses are perfect for serving tall, cool, drinks in style.

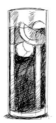

Old-Fashioned Glass

The old-fashioned glass, also known as a rocks glass, is a short, squat tumbler and is great for a smaller beverage with a classy garnish.

Champagne Flute

The tall, thin flute's tapered design helps keep fizz in a drink longer.

Margarita Glass

This wide-rimmed glass, as its name indicates, is used to serve blended ice drinks or creamy frozen beverages.

oupe Glass

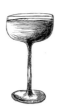

other wide-rimmed
ss that is good for
ving sparkling drinks
l an elegant alternative
he martini glass.

ifter Glass

e bowl-shaped snifter
ss, also referred to as a
oon, invites drinkers
radle the drink in their
ds, warming the contents
he glass, so it is a good
ion for warmed mocktails,
h as a mulled mock wine.
e aroma of the drink is
d in the glass, allowing
to breathe in the drink's
ma before sipping it.

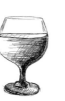

urricane Glass

is pear-shaped glass pays
mage to the hurricane
p. It is the glass used
create the New Orleans
m-based cocktail, the
rricane. It's also an
ellent glass for a variety of
zen and blended mocktails.

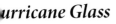

Pitcher

Although not strictly a glass,
a pitcher or jug is a great
addition to your mocktail
glassware. Mocktails are
perfect drinks to be shared
with friends and family
and a good pitcher is an
easy way to ensure there
is enough for everyone.

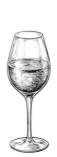

Wine Glass

The style of wine glass we see
today is closely related to the
Jacobite glass used to drink
wine from the 1700s onwards,
on which each Freemason
lodge had their own design
engraved. Today there is a
huge variety of wine glasses,
most off them stemmed
to keep the drink cold.

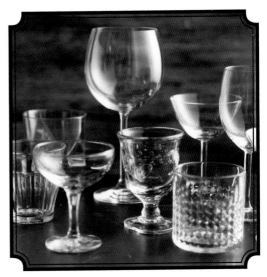

EQUIPMENT

The equipment you have in your home bar will depend on whether you are someone who likes all the latest gadgets, or whether you are happy making do with some basic options. There is no limit to the amount of bar equipment available, but you don't need lots of gadgets to make most of the drinks in this book. Here are the essential tools of the trade.

Jigger

A jigger is a bartender's basic measuring tool and essential for crafting the perfect blend of ingredients. It usually has a measurement on each end, such as 1 ounce and 1½ ounces. Get a steel jigger with clear measurement markings so you can easily and accurately pour out measures.

Shaker

Most contemporary shakers are made from steel as steel doesn't tarnish readily and doesn't conduct heat easily—this is useful when making chilled mocktails as the ice cools the mocktail rather than the shaker. Most standard shakers, known as cobbler shakers, come with a built-in strainer, but if you're using a Boston or Parisian shaker then you'll need to use a separate strainer.

Barspoon

A barspoon has a small bowl and a long handle that allows you to muddle, mix, and stir with ease. Spoons come in a variety of lengths and widths. A stylishly designed barspoon is an attractive addition to any bartender's kit.

Strainer

A Hawthorne strainer is an essential tool to prevent ice and other ingredients being poured into your glass. Some mocktails need to be double-strained so even if there is a strainer in your cocktail shaker, you'll still need a separate fine strainer in your bar collection. Another style of strainer is the julep strainer, used to hold ice back in stirred drinks.

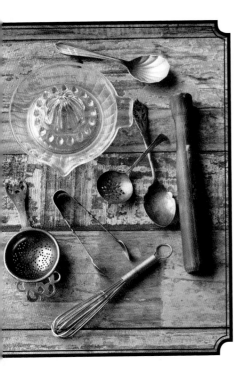

Juicer

A traditional, ridged half-lemon shape on a saucer will work perfectly well for juicing small amounts. There is also a citrus spout that screws into a lemon or lime and is useful for obtaining tiny amounts of juice. Mechanical or electric presses are great for large amounts of juice, but are not essential in a home bar. A less expensive option is called a hand juicer—these work by pressing the juice out of citrus fruits.

Other Equipment

Other items you might need for your home bar are olive sticks, blender, tongs, an ice bucket, a chopping board, knives, jugs, straws, and an espuma gun for making foams.

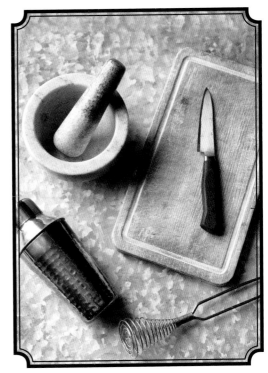

ixing Glass

y vessel that holds about 2 cups of liquid be used for mixing drinks. It is good nave a mixing glass with a spout or ged rim so that you can stop ice from ping into the glass. Mixing beakers increasingly popular nowadays, and usually made of glass or crystal.

uddler

mashing up citrus fruit or crushing herbs, need a muddler. This is a chunky wooden metal tool with a rounded end and it can o be used to make cracked ice. You can sh fruit or crush herbs with a mortar and stle, but the advantage of a muddler is that an be used directly in the mixing glass.

TERMS & TECHNIQUES

Shaking and stirring are the two most basic mixology techniques, and are essential to master to make a delicious mocktail. The other techniques described here—building, layering, muddling, blending, creating foams and airs, and infusing—all add to your repertoire of bartender's techniques.

Shaking and Stirring

Shaking is when you add all the ingredients, including ice cubes, to the shaker and shake vigorously until well chilled. The benefits of shaking are that the drink is rapidly mixed, chilled, and aerated. Once the drink has been shaken, the outside of the shaker should be lightly frosted.

Shaking a mocktail will dilute your drink quite significantly. This gives recipes the correct balance of taste and temperature. The drink is then double-strained into glasses—the shaker could have a built-in strainer and you usually use a separate strainer over the glass as well. Shaking is also used to prepare mocktails that include an ingredient that will not combine with less vigorous forms of mixing, such as egg white.

Stirring is the purist's choice, a mixing technique where you combine all the ingredients, usually with some ice cubes, in a mixing glass and stir them together using a long-handled barspoon or swizzle stick. This allows you to blend and chill the ingredients without too much erosion of the ice, so you can control the level of dilution.

Building and Layering

Building involves the pouring of all the ingredients, one by one, usually over ice, into the serving glass. You might then stir the mocktail briefly to mix it rather than to chill or aerate it. You need to follow built recipes exactly, as the order of the ingredients can vary and this can affect the flavor.

Layering requires concentration, precision and a steady hand. To make layered mocktails, you generally pour the heaviest liquid first, working through to the lightest. However, the real trick is the technique. Either touch the top of the drink with a long-handled barspoon and pour the liquid slowly over the back of it to disperse it across the top of the ingredients already in the glass, or pour the liquid down the twisted stem that many barspoons have. You should hold the spoon's flat disc just above the drink. Use a clean barspoon for each layer. Floating is the term used to describe adding the top layer.

Muddling and Blending

Muddling is the extraction of the juice or oils from the pulp or skin of a fruit, herb or spice. It involves mashing ingredients to release their flavors and it is usually done with a large pestle-like implement called a muddler.

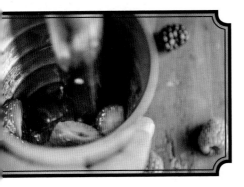

An air is an extremely light froth with an effervescent texture that is less heavy than a foam—the texture can range from a bubble bath foam to a light fizz. To make a light air, the best ingredient to use is lecithin. Whisk a pinch of powdered lecithin with simple syrup using a hand whisk or electric mixer until you have a light air. If you prefer a finer air, use a milk frother.

e end of the muddler that is used to crush redients is thicker, flatter and sometimes ked. The best muddling technique is to keep ssing down with a twisting action until the redient has released all its oil or juice. You also use a pestle and mortar or the end wooden spoon.

nding is when all mocktail ingredients combined in a blender or food processor. is is used when mixing ingredients such whole fruit, or with creamy ingredients t do not combine well unless they are nded. These drinks are often blended h crushed or cracked ice to produce cktails with a smooth, frozen consistency.

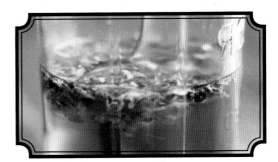

ams and Airs

ms and airs can be created in various cknesses, from a light froth to a heavy, amy foam. For a simple foam, use egg white, on juice and sugar—to top two mocktails, t whisk 1 egg white, ½ ounce of lemon juice 1 teaspoon of superfine sugar together until roughly mixed. This mixture can then be ced into an espuma gun or cream whipper, rged, shaken and sprayed over the top of mocktails for a light, creamy finish. The sher the egg white, the more stable the foam.

Infusions

Infusions allow you to combine flavors to produce some inventive new ingredients. When you make a cup of tea, the tea leaves change the color and taste of the water they have infused. It is the same with mixed drinks. You can infuse water, syrups, juices, and even condiments. To infuse flavors, you need to steep them in your choice of ingredient for a minimum of 24 hours. When the right strength of flavor has imparted, the solids are strained out. The infused ingredient can then be stored in the fridge for up to 2 weeks.

Creating infusions means that you will always have flavored mixtures to hand, instead of having to muddle ingredients each time. The depth of flavor should be strong, depending on how long the infusions have been left to mix.

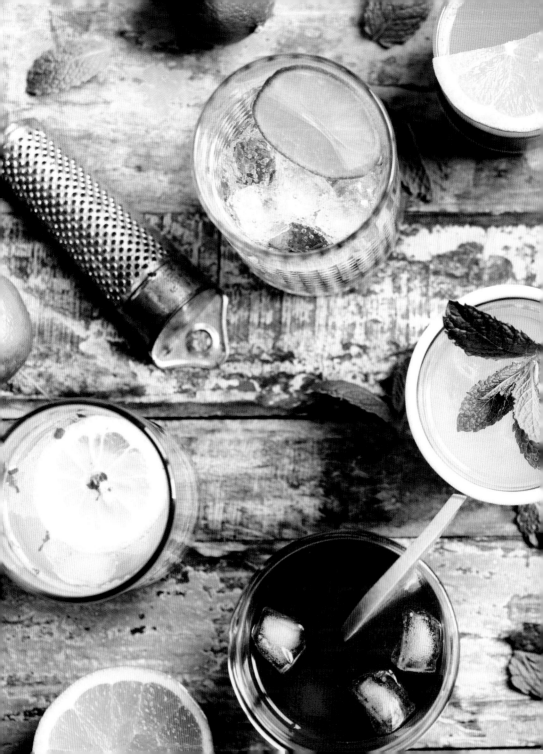

Chapter 1

FRESH

These mocktails immerse themselves in nature's bounty and in the cool and refreshing—here we embrace apples, pears, mint, rosewater, crisp produce, pure ingredients, and hydrating, uplifting combinations.

LAVENDER LEMONADE

Serves 1

Ingredients

9 ounces boiling water

¼ ounce dried lavender

2¾ ounces sugar

2 ounces fresh lemon juice

5 ounces chilled sparkling water

lavender sprig, to garnish

1. Put the boiling water into a small pan or heatproof bowl and add the lavender. Then add the sugar and stir to dissolve.

2. Cover and leave in the refrigerator overnight to infuse.

3. Strain into a clean bottle and store in the refrigerator.

4. Fill a highball glass with ice cubes and add 2 ounces of the lavender syrup. Add the lemon juice and stir to mix.

5. Top with sparkling water and garnish with a lavender sprig.

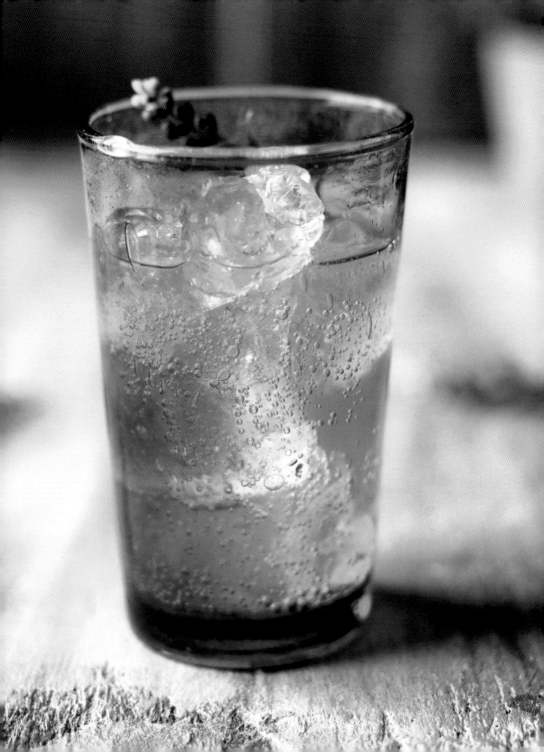

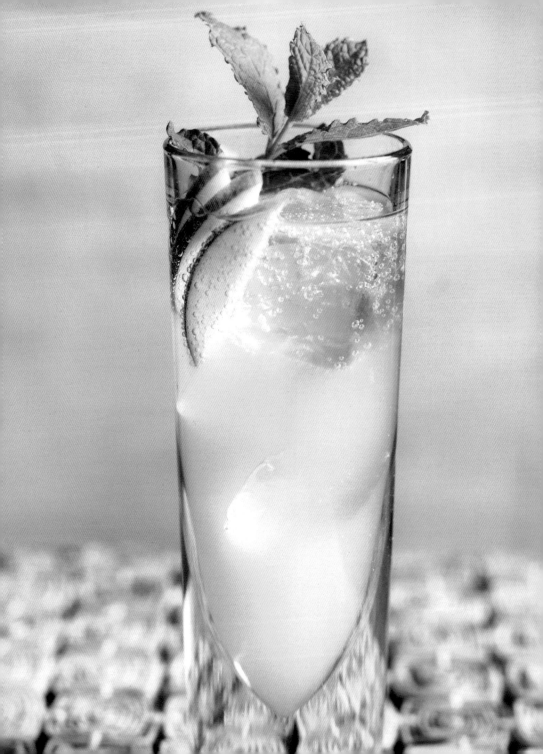

APPLE MINT CHILL

Serves 1

Ingredients

4 teaspoons elderflower cordial

2 tablespoons fresh lemon juice

4 ounces unfiltered apple juice

6 fresh mint leaves

3½ tablespoons soda water

fresh mint sprig, to garnish

apple fan, to garnish

1. Fill a highball glass with ice cubes and add the cordial, lemon juice, and apple juice. Stir well to mix.

2. Bruise the mint, add to the glass and stir again.

3. Top with soda water, garnish with the mint sprig and an apple fan.

VANILLA ICED TEA

Serves 1

Ingredients

2 teaspoons fresh lemon juice

3 fresh mint leaves

4 ounces cold breakfast tea
or peppermint tea

fresh mint sprig, to garnish

lemon wheel, to garnish

Vanilla Syrup

1 split vanilla bean

bottle agave syrup

1. Add the split vanilla bean to the bottle of agave syrup and leave it in the bottle to infuse overnight.. The pod can stay in the bottle as you use the infused agave.

2. Put the lemon juice and 2 teaspoons of the syrup into the base of a rocks glass and stir to dissolve the agave.

3. Crush the mint leaves and add to the glass.

4. Fill the glass with ice cubes and pour over the tea.

5. Stir well to mix and garnish with a mint sprig and lemon wheel.

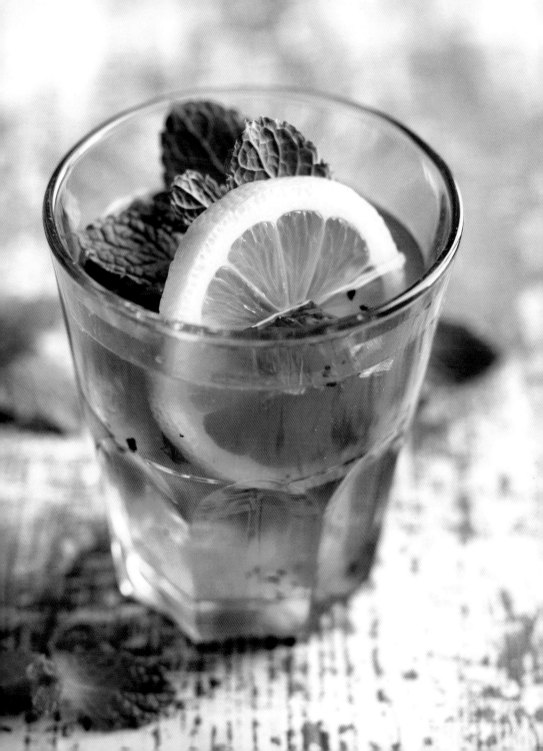

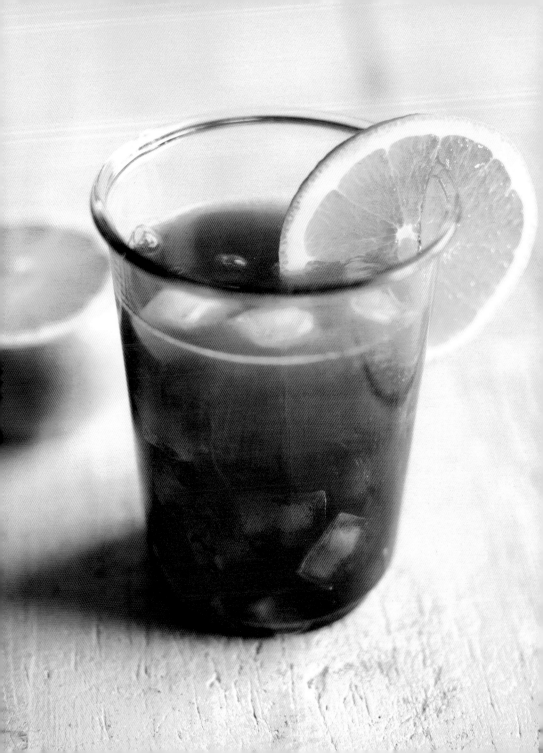

SHIRLEY TEMPLE

Serves 1

Ingredients

1½ ounces lemon juice

¾ ounce grenadine

ginger ale

orange slice, to garnish

1. Put 4–6 ice cubes into a cocktail shaker.

2. Pour over the lemon juice and grenadine and shake vigorously until well frosted.

3. Fill a chilled glass halfway with ice, then strain the liquid over it.

4. Top up with ginger ale and garnish with the orange slice.

PROHIBITION PUNCH

Serves 12

Ingredients

24 ounces apple juice

12 ounces lemon juice

4 ounces simple syrup

64 ounces ginger ale

orange slices, to garnish

1. Pour the apple juice into a large pitcher.

2. Add the lemon juice and simple syrup and a handful of ice cubes.

3. Add the ginger ale and stir gently to mix.

4. Pour into chilled lowball glasses and garnish with orange slices.

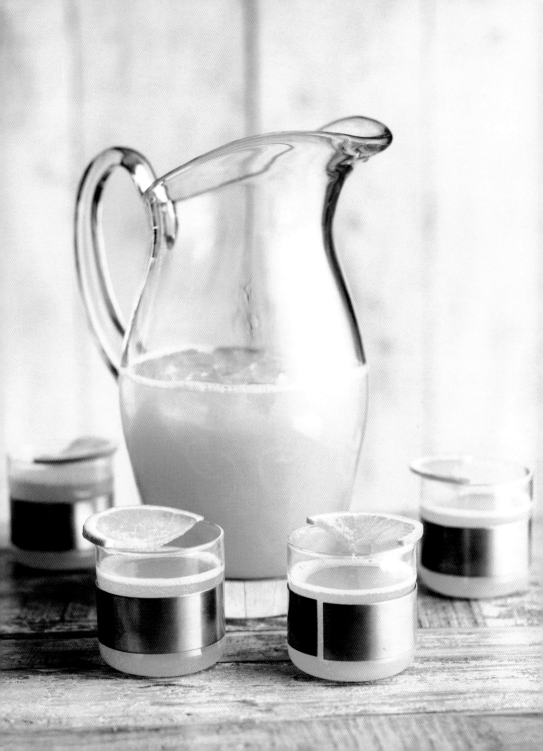

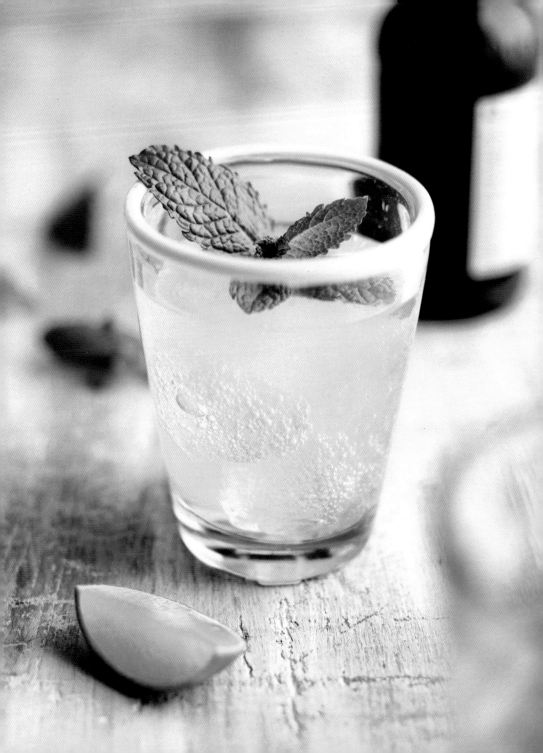

LONG BOAT

Serves 1

Ingredients

1½ ounces sweetened lime juice

ginger beer

lime wedge, to garnish

fresh mint sprig, to garnish

1. Fill a chilled glass two-thirds full with ice and pour in the sweetened lime juice.

2. Top up with ginger beer and stir gently.

3. Garnish with the lime wedge and the mint sprig.

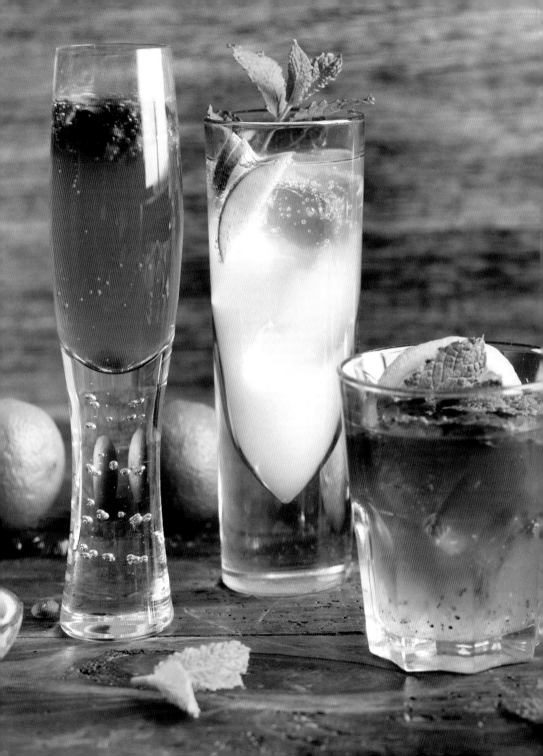

THE BENEFITS OF
MOCKTAILS

Drinking mocktails has significant advantages over drinking alcohol. To begin with, any type of alcohol comes at a price. Because mocktails are nonalcoholic, they are naturally less expensive.

Alcoholic drinks and sugary mixed drinks can add copious calories to your daily allowance. The average mixed drink with a single shot of spirit with high sugar content, juice, or flavored soda totals around 200 calories. Multiply that by two or three over the course of an evening and you will have to run an extra hour to burn it off. Mocktails made with fresh fruit, sensible syrups, and edible garnishes can come in at around half or less of this calorie value.

Mocktails also generally have more nutrients than cocktails. Those made with fresh and/or organic juices, such as pomegranate, mango, and cranberry, boast plenty of antioxidants and vitamin C. Drinks containing these ingredients also mean that you will be consuming natural sugars.

Finally, mocktails can be enjoyed by everyone—designated drivers, pregnant people, people on medication or with chronic illnesses, children, and the most devout teetotalers. This makes for a more inclusive atmosphere at a party or other event where everyone can have an interesting choice of drinks.

POMEGRANATE & ROSE SLUSHY

Serves 8-10

Ingredients

8 fresh mint sprigs, to garnish (optional)

sparkling or still water, to serve

Pomegranate and Rose Syrup

juice of 2 lemons

¼ teaspoon rosewater

7 ounces fresh pomegranate juice (juice of about 2 pomegranates)

7 ounces superfine sugar

1. To make the syrup, put the lemon juice, rosewater, pomegranate juice, and sugar in a saucepan, stir and cook over a low heat until the sugar has dissolved.

2. Increase the heat to medium-high, bring to a boil, then reduce the heat to low and simmer for 3–4 minutes. Boiling sugar is very hot, so handle with care and make sure it doesn't bubble over. Leave to cool completely.

3. Put some crushed ice in a tall glass. Pour a dash of the syrup over the ice and add a sprig of mint, if using. Pour in still or sparkling water to taste, mix well and serve immediately.

4. The syrup will keep in the refrigerator in a sealed container for 3–4 days.

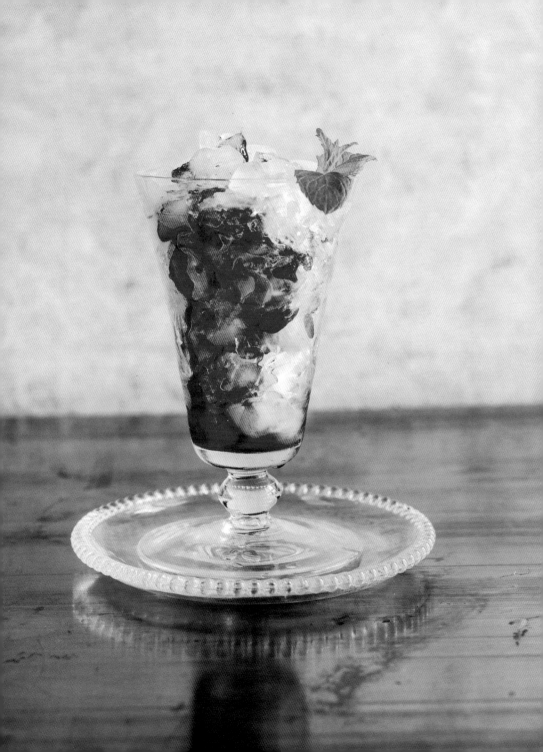

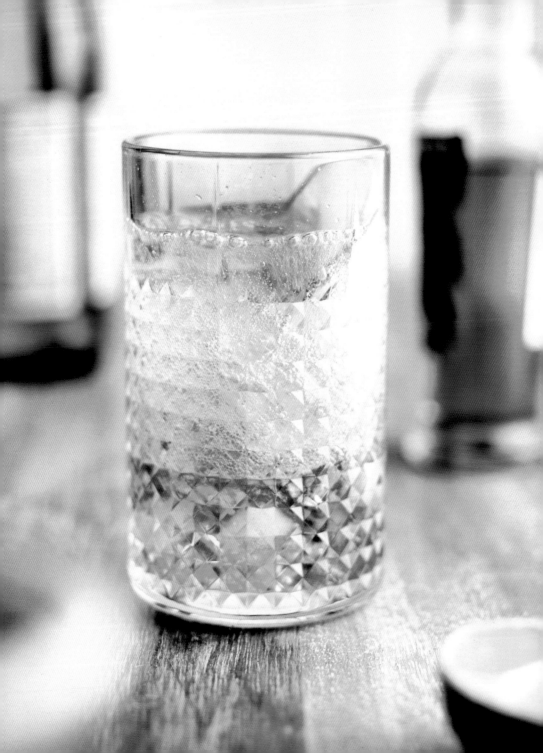

ITALIAN SODA

Serves 1

Ingredients

2¼ ounces hazelnut syrup

sparkling water

lime slice, to garnish

1. Fill a chilled Collins glass with ice.

2. Pour the hazelnut syrup over and fill with sparkling water. Stir gently and dress with a slice of lime.

ARNOLD PALMER

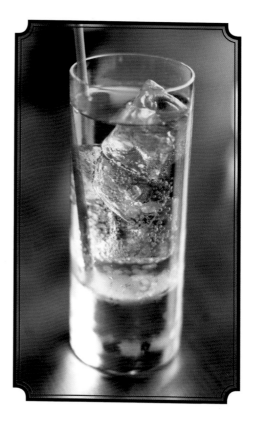

Serves 1

—

Ingredients

4½ ounces lemonade

4½ ounces iced tea

1. Half fill a chilled highball glass with ice cubes and pour in the lemonade.

2. Slowly pour in the tea, so that it does not mix.

3. Serve immediately with a straw.

VIRGIN GINGER FIZZ

Serves 1

—

Ingredients

ginger ale

3 fresh mint sprigs

fresh raspberries, to garnish

fresh mint sprig, to garnish

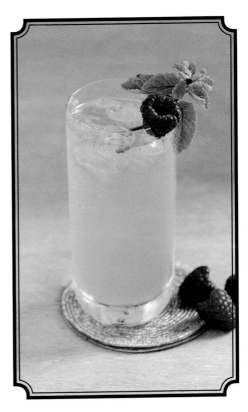

1. Put 3 ounces of ginger ale into a blender.

2. Add the mint sprigs and blend together.

3. Strain into a chilled highball glass that is two-thirds filled with ice. Top up with more ginger ale.

4. Garnish with raspberries and the mint sprig.

VIRGIN BITTER GUNNER

Serves 1

—

Ingredients

2 ounces lime juice

2 teaspoons nonalcoholic
aromatic bitters, or to taste

3½ ounces ginger beer

3½ ounces lemonade

lime slice, to garnish

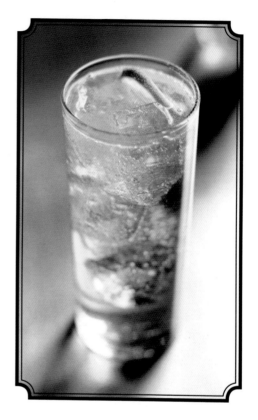

1. Mix all the ingredients together in a highball glass.

2. Taste and add more bitters if you wish.

3. Add the lime slice to the glass.

SALTY PUPPY

Serves 1

—

Ingredients

1 teaspoon granulated sugar

1 teaspoon kosher salt

lime wedge

¾ ounce lime juice

grapefruit juice

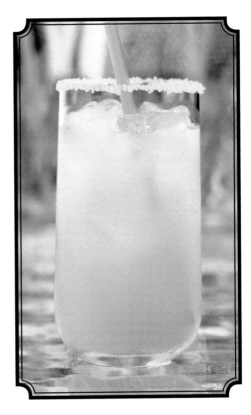

1. Mix the sugar and salt together on a saucer.

2. Rub the rim of a chilled highball glass with the lime wedge and twist the glass rim into the sugar and salt mixture to frost.

3. Fill the glass with ice and add the lime juice.
Top with grapefruit juice.

VIRGIN COLLINS

Serves 1

Ingredients

6 fresh mint leaves,
plus extra to garnish

1 teaspoon superfine sugar

3 ounces lemon juice

sparkling water

lemon slice, to garnish

1. Put the mint leaves
into a chilled Collins
or highball glass.

2. Add the sugar
and lemon juice.

3. Muddle the mint
leaves and stir until the
sugar has dissolved.

4. Fill the glass with ice cubes
and top with sparkling water.
Stir gently and garnish with
the fresh mint and lemon slice.

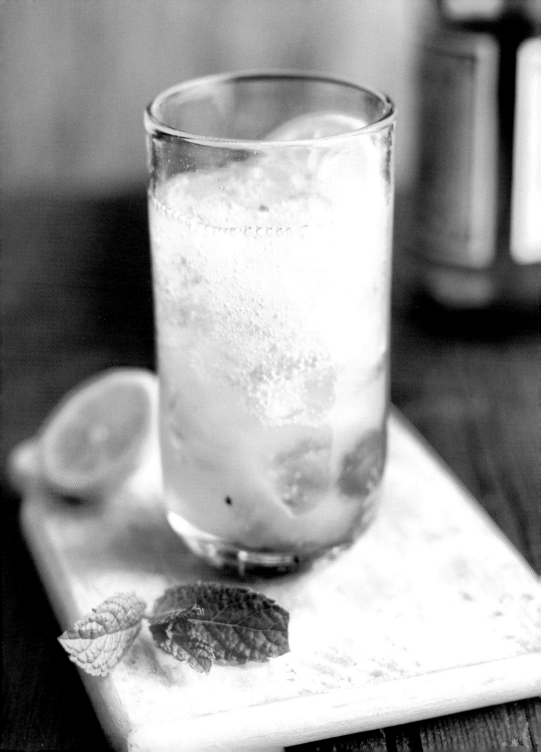

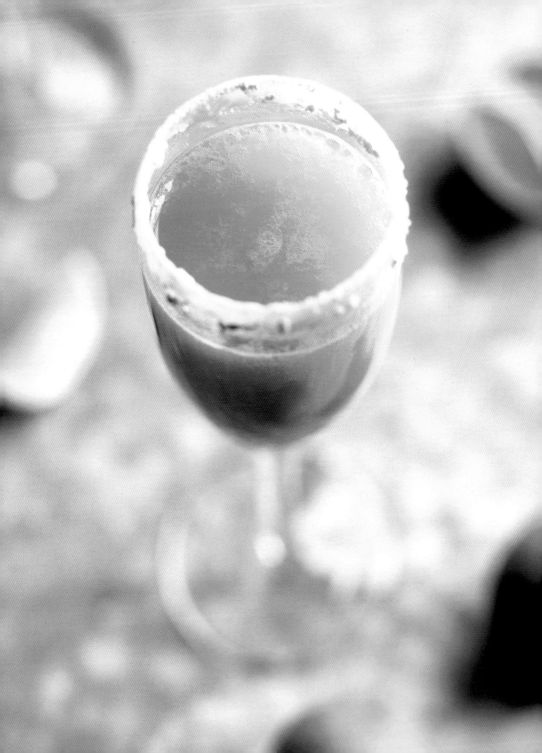

ORANGE & LIME FIZZ

Serves 1

Ingredients

3 ounces chilled fresh orange juice

confectioners' sugar

juice of half a lime

few drops nonalcoholic aromatic bitters

3–4½ ounces sparkling water

1. Rub the rim of a flute with orange or lime juice and dip into the confectioners' sugar.

2. Stir the rest of the juices together with the bitters and then pour into the glass.

3. Add sparkling water to taste.

GRAPEFRUIT COOLER

Serves 6

Ingredients

2 ounces fresh mint

3 ounces simple syrup

16 ounces grapefruit juice

6 ounces lemon juice

sparkling water

fresh mint sprigs, to garnish

1. Muddle fresh mint leaves in a small bowl with the simple syrup.

2. Set aside for at least 2 hours to steep, mashing again from time to time.

3. Strain the steeped mixture into a pitcher and add the grapefruit juice and lemon juice. Cover with plastic wrap and chill for at least 2 hours.

4. To serve, fill six chilled Collins glasses with ice. Divide the grapefruit mixture evenly in the glasses, then top with sparkling water. Garnish with fresh mint.

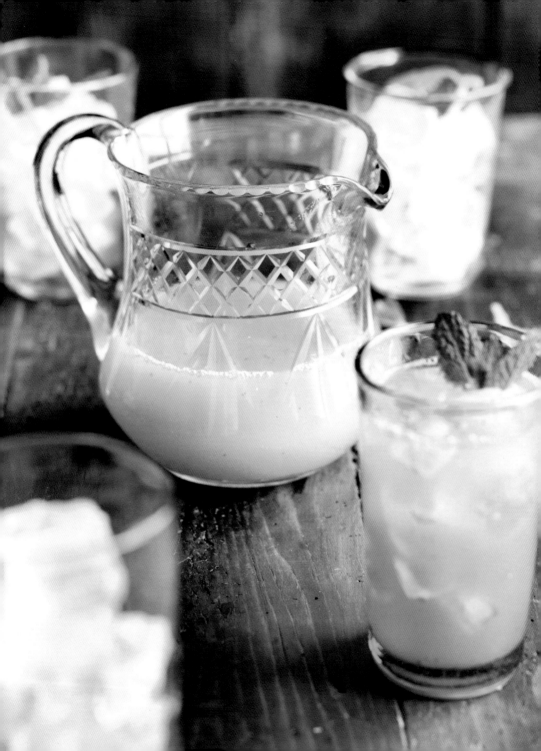

HONEYDEW COOLER

Serves 2

—

Ingredients

9 ounces honeydew melon

10 ounces sparkling water

2 tablespoons honey

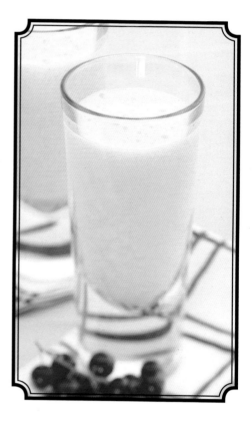

1. Cut the rind off the melon. Chop the melon into chunks, discarding any seeds.

2. Put into a food processor with the water and honey and process until smooth. Pour into glasses.

APPLE FRAZZLE

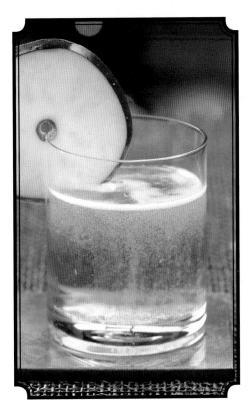

Serves 1

—

Ingredients

6 ounces apple juice

1 teaspoon simple syrup

½ teaspoon lemon juice

sparkling water

apple slice, to garnish

1. Shake the apple juice, simple syrup, and lemon juice vigorously over ice until well frosted.

2. Strain into a chilled tumbler and top with sparkling water.
Garnish with a slice of apple.

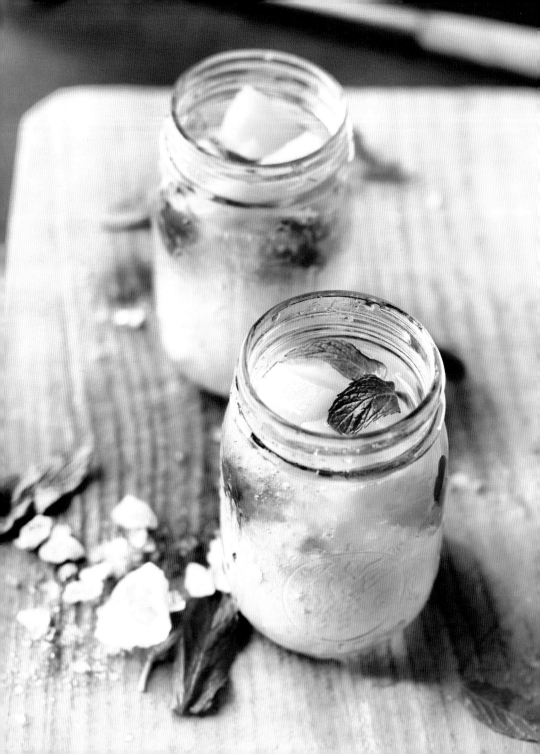

PINEAPPLE & MINT ICED TEA

Serves 4

Ingredients

1 pineapple

3½ cups water

1 ounce fresh mint

2-inch piece of fresh ginger, peeled and finely sliced

4 ounces agave syrup

2 tablespoons fresh mint leaves, to garnish

1. Prepare the pineapple by slicing off the base and leaves with a sharp knife. Rest the pineapple on its base and slice off the peel, until you reveal the flesh. Slice the fruit in half and remove the woody core that sits down the center. Cut the remaining flesh into ¾-inch cubes. Reserve 8 cubes for use later.

2. Pour the water into a large saucepan and add the pineapple, mint, and ginger. Stir in the agave syrup and place the saucepan over a medium-high heat. Simmer for 45 minutes, or until the liquid has reduced by half.

3. Remove from the heat and allow the nectar to cool completely and infuse. This will take 4–5 hours. Using a slotted spoon, remove the mint sprigs and ginger.

4. Add ice, mint leaves, and reserved pineapple cubes to the bottom of a large pitcher. Pour over the cooled nectar and stir to mix.

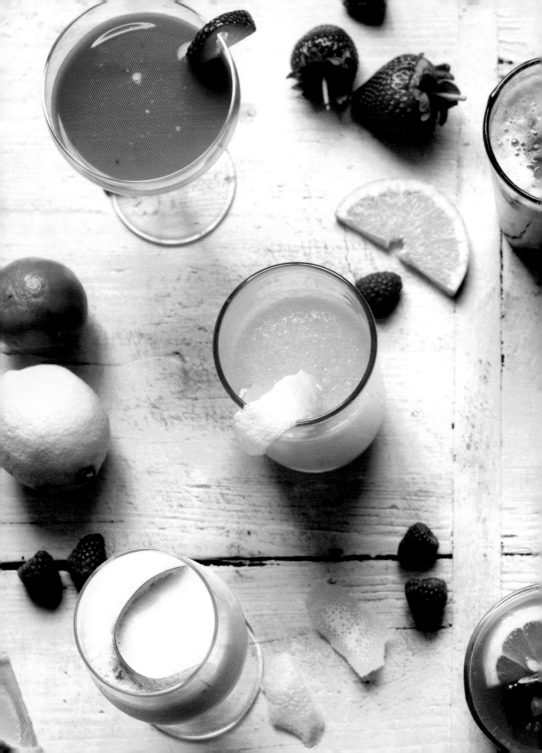

Chapter 2
ZING

Here are mocktails with citrus flavors and reviving combinations.
Discover the tang of lemon, orange, grapefruit, and lime, and
the clean-cut tastes of pomegranate, grape, and ginger, finished
with citrus peel curls, orange slices, and lime wedges.

QUEEN OF GREENS

Serves 1

Ingredients

4 kale leaves, stems included

6 fresh mint leaves

4 teaspoons ginger syrup

2 tablespoons fresh lime juice

fresh mint sprig, to garnish

1. Juice the kale leaves using a juicer or a blender.

2. Fill a cocktail shaker with ice cubes, add the kale juice, mint leaves, ginger syrup, and lime juice. Shake vigorously for 15 seconds.

3. Put 4–5 ice cubes into a large wine glass and strain the mocktail over it.

4. Garnish with mint sprig.

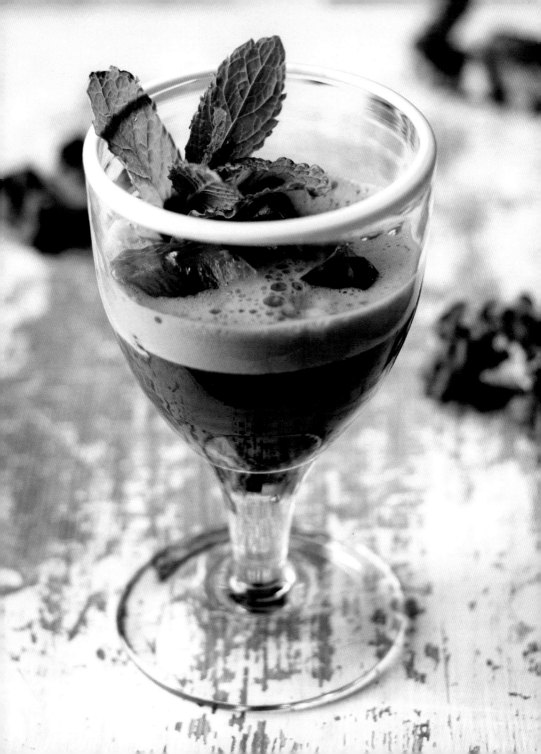

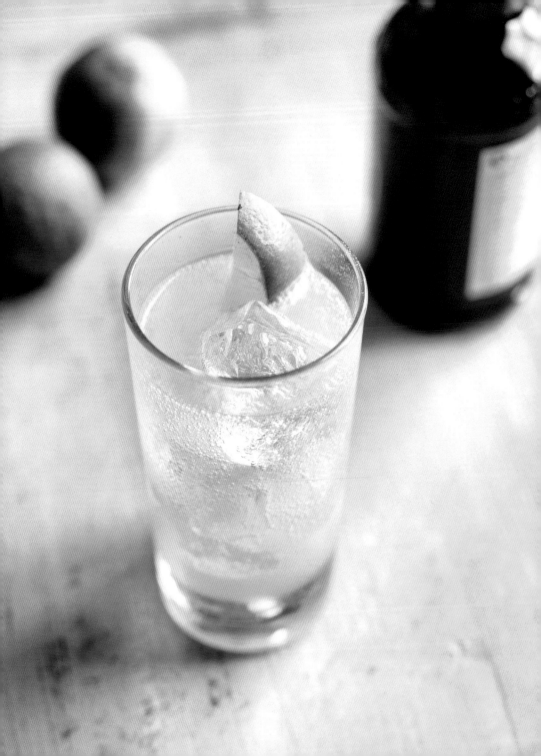

SAINT KIDD

Serves 1

Ingredients

2 teaspoons apple pie syrup

1 tablespoon fresh lime juice

3½ ounces apple juice

2 ounces ginger beer

lime wedge, to garnish

1. Fill a highball glass with ice cubes and add the syrup.

2. Add the lime and apple juice, stir well, and top with the ginger beer.

3. Garnish with the lime wedge.

PINK FIZZ

Serves 1

Ingredients

5 teaspoons
pomegranate juice, chilled

4 ounces ginger ale, chilled

1 teaspoon pomegranate seeds,
to garnish

1. Pour the pomegranate
juice into a champagne flute.

2. Top with chilled ginger ale.

3. Garnish with the
pomegranate seeds.

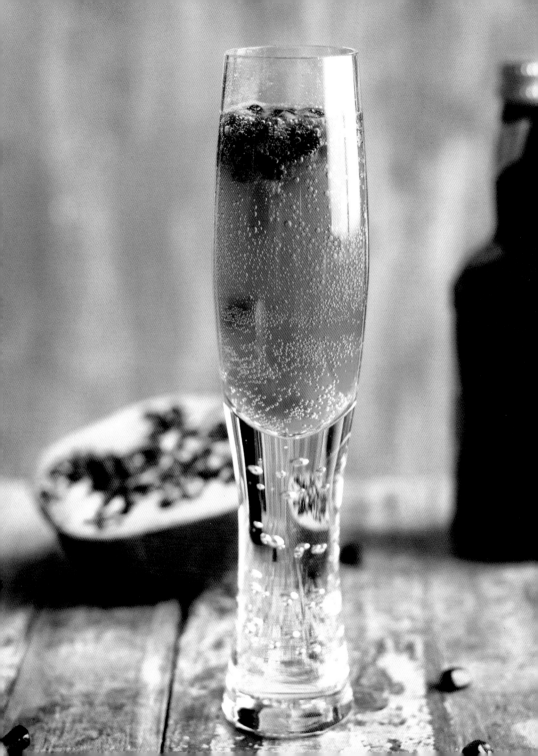

LEMON FIZZ

Serves 1

—

Ingredients

2 fresh lemons

peel of ½ lemon

1 tablespoon sugar

sparkling lemonade, chilled

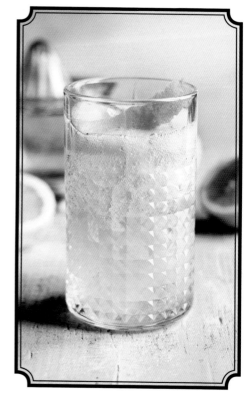

1. Squeeze the fresh lemons and pour the juice into a chilled highball glass filled with crushed ice.

2. Add the lemon peel and sugar to taste and stir briefly.

3. Top with lemonade to taste.

ST. CLEMENTS

Serves 1

—

Ingredients

3 ounces orange juice

3 ounces bitter lemon

orange and lemon slices,
to garnish

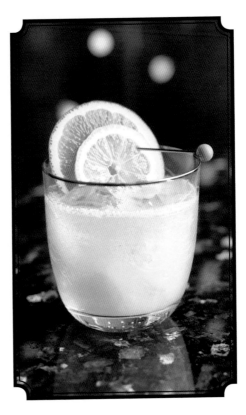

1. Add ice cubes to a chilled tumbler.
Pour in the orange juice and bitter lemon.

2. Stir gently and garnish with orange and lemon slices.

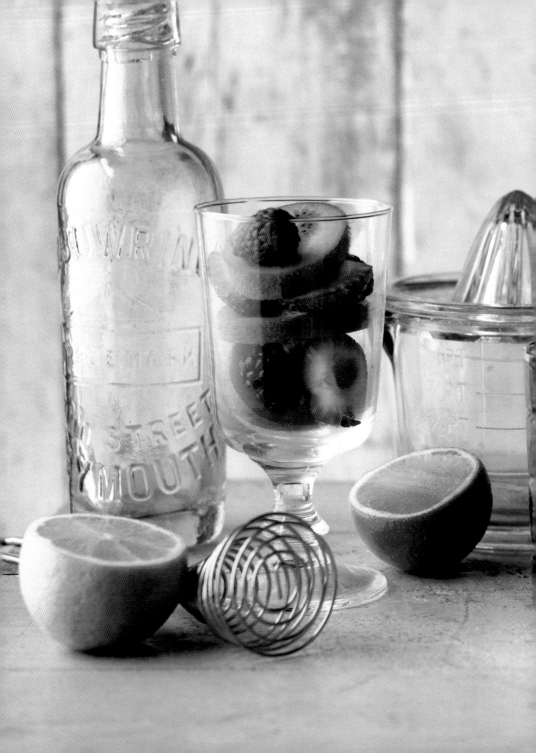

FRESH IS
BEST

Many mocktail recipes call for fresh juices, but what does this really mean? And why are fresh juices better than cartons of juice from a store? Essentially, a fresh juice is one that is juiced or squeezed directly from the fruit without any processing. Using freshly squeezed fruit juices has significant benefits, both to the flavor of your mocktails and to your physical health. Fresh homemade juices contain more vitamins, minerals, and nutritional compounds, such as enzymes and flavonoids, than commercial juices, which lose their goodness over time and may contain added sugar.

Fresh fruit and vegetable juices can also assist with digestion. This is because a liquid is easier to digest than solids, so your digestive system doesn't have to work so hard. The soluble fiber in fresh juices can also help lower cholesterol.

Although you might think that squeezing fresh juice is a time-consuming job, drinking it can help you preserve your energy stores. Our bodies use energy to convert the foods we eat into a liquid state ready to be absorbed. When you drink fresh juice, your body essentially skips this step and saves energy. This is the reason that your body feels revived after a healthy meal and at a low ebb after eating junk food.

NONALCOHOLIC PIMM'S

Serves 6

Ingredients

16 ounces lemonade, chilled

15 ounces cola, chilled

15 ounces dry ginger ale, chilled

juice of 1 orange

juice of 1 lemon

few drops nonalcoholic
aromatic bitters

sliced fruit, such as apples,
strawberries, and oranges

fresh mint sprigs

1. Mix the first six ingredients together thoroughly in a large pitcher or punch bowl.

2. Float in the fruit and mint. Keep the Pimm's in a cold place and add the ice cubes just before serving.

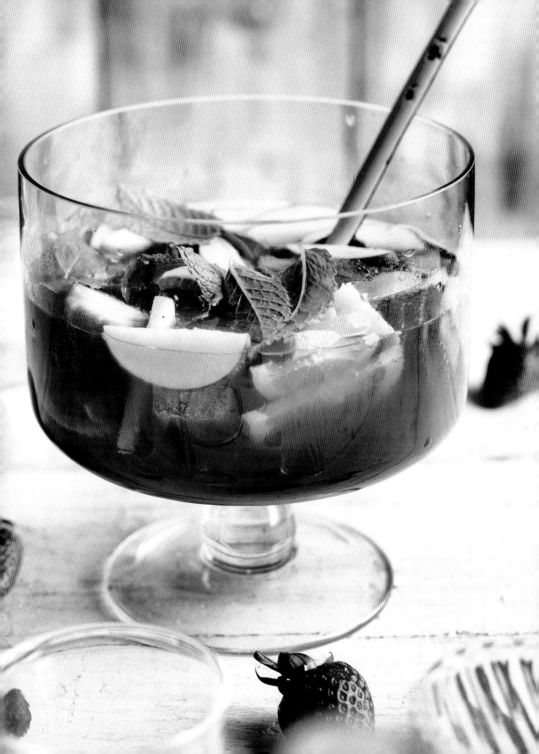

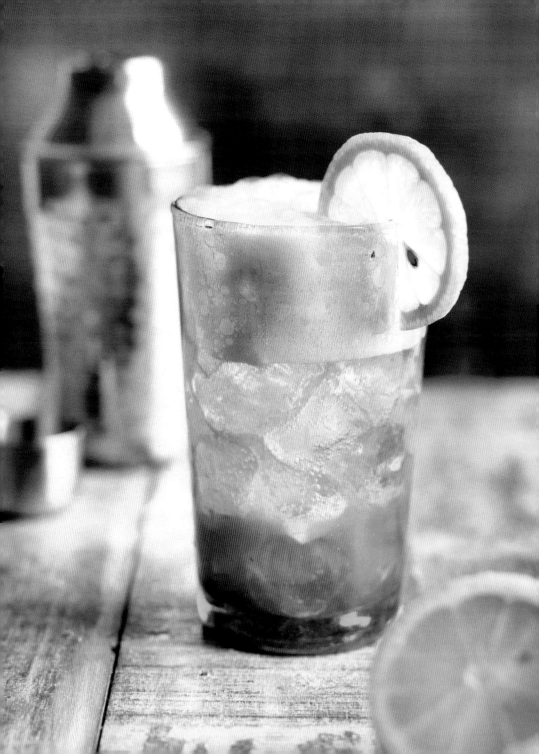

POM POM

Serves 1

Ingredients

juice of ½ lemon

1 egg white

1 dash grenadine

lemonade

lemon slice, to garnish

1. Shake the lemon juice, egg white, and grenadine together and strain over the ice cubes in a tall glass.

2. Top with lemonade and garnish with a lemon slice on the rim of the glass.

PINKY PINK

Serves 1

Ingredients

1½ ounces lemon juice

1½ ounces orange juice

2–3 strawberries, mashed

1½ ounces strawberry syrup

½ egg yolk

1 dash grenadine

orange slice, to garnish

1. Place the lemon juice, orange juice, strawberries, strawberry syrup, egg yolk, and grenadine in a cocktail shaker and add ice cubes. Shake vigorously.

2. Strain the mixture into a cocktail glass and garnish with the orange slice.

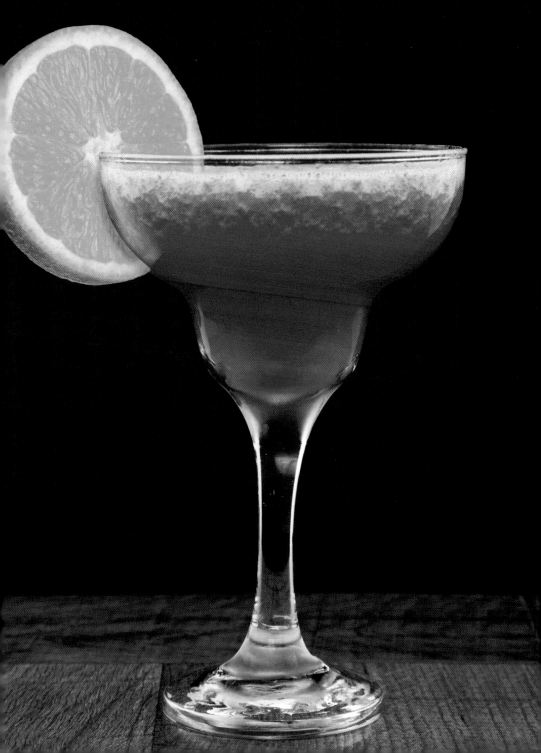

MAIDENLY MIMOSA

Serves 2

—

Ingredients

6 ounces orange juice

6 ounces sparkling
white grape juice

orange slices, to garnish

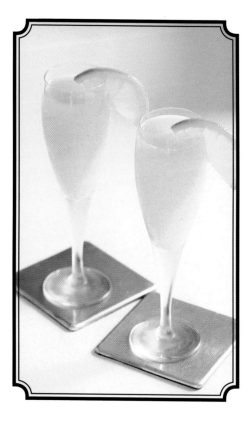

1. Chill two champagne flutes.

2. Divide the orange juice between the flutes and top with the sparkling grape juice.

3. Garnish with the orange slices.

SLUSH PUPPY

Serves 1

—

Ingredients

juice of 1 lemon or
½ pink grapefruit

1 ounce grenadine

zest of ½ lemon

2–3 teaspoons
raspberry syrup

soda water

maraschino cherry,
to garnish

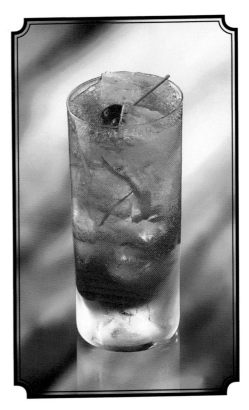

1. Pour the lemon or grapefruit juice juice and grenadine
into a chilled tall Collins glass with ice.

2. Add the lemon zest, syrup, and soda water to taste.
Garnish with cherry.

LITTLE PRINCE

Serves 1

—

Ingredients

1½ ounces apricot juice

1½ ounces lemon juice

3 ounces sparkling
apple juice

lemon peel twist, to garnish

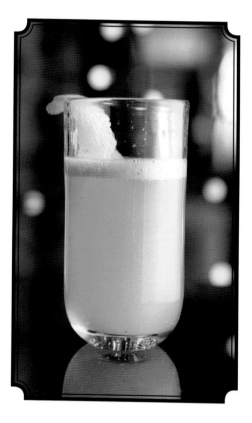

1. Add ice to a mixing glass. Pour the apricot juice,
lemon juice, and apple juice over the ice and stir well.

2. Strain into a chilled highball glass and dress with a lemon twist.

BLOOD ORANGE ON THE TRACKS

Serves 1

—

Ingredients

¾ ounce
nonalcoholic bitters

3¾ ounces blood
orange juice

sparkling water

orange slice, to garnish

fresh mint sprig, to garnish

1. Pour the bitters into a chilled highball glass filled with ice.

2. Add the blood orange juice. Do not stir.

3. Top with sparkling water.

4. Garnish with the orange slice and mint.

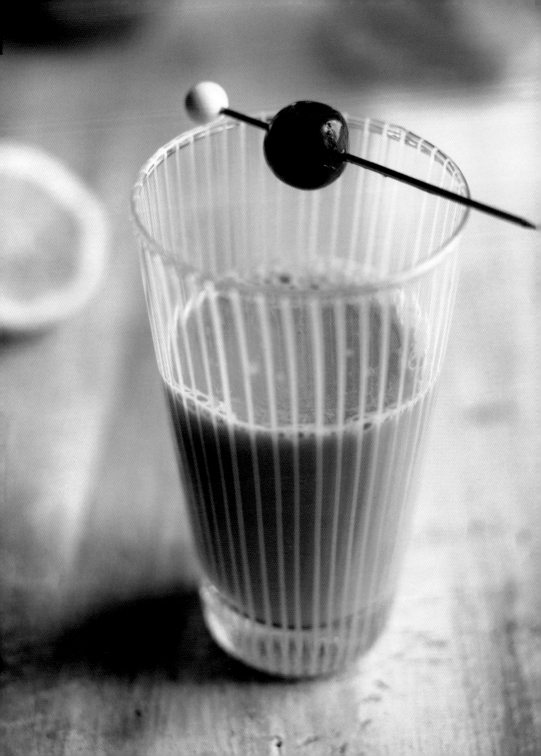

PARSON'S PARTICULAR

Serves 1

Ingredients

3 ounces fresh orange juice

1½ ounces fresh lemon juice

1 egg yolk

4 dashes grenadine

marachino cherry, to garnish

1. Shake all the ingredients together over ice until well frosted and strain into a Collins glass.

2. Garnish with a cocktail cherry.

APPLE SOUR

Serves 1

Ingredients

6 ounces apple juice

juice of 1 lemon

juice of 1 lime

1½ ounces honey

1 egg white

4–5 raspberries

long apple peel strip, to garnish

1. Blend the apple juice, lemon and lime juices, honey, and egg white with ice in a blender until frothy and slushy.

2. Put the raspberries in the bottom of a chilled glass, crush with a wooden spoon, and pour in the fruit slush.

3. Garnish with a strip of apple peel.

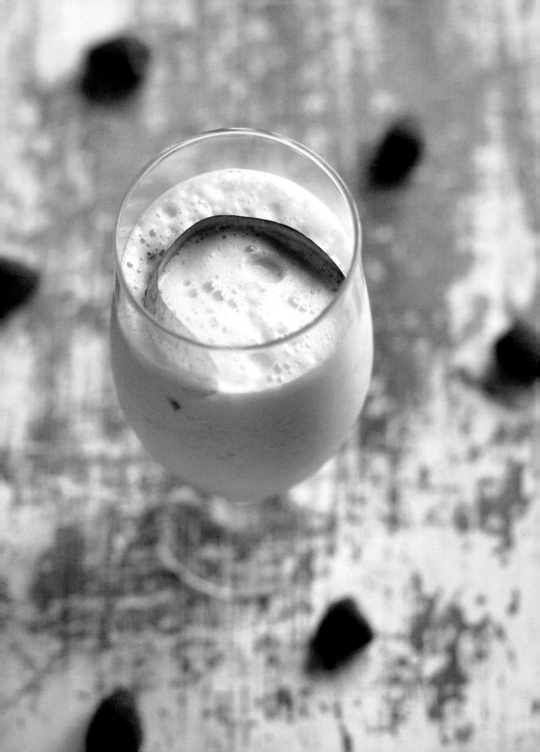

RED APPLE SUNSET

Serves 1

—

Ingredients

3 ounces apple juice

3 ounces grapefruit juice

1 dash grenadine

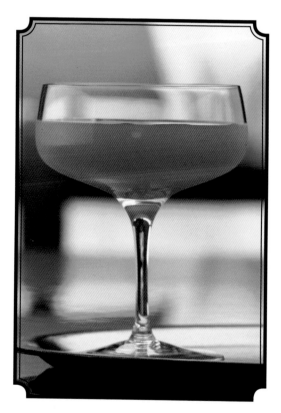

1. Shake the apple juice, grapefruit juice, and dash of grenadine over ice cubes until well frosted.

2. Strain into a chilled cocktail glass.

SOBER SUNDAY

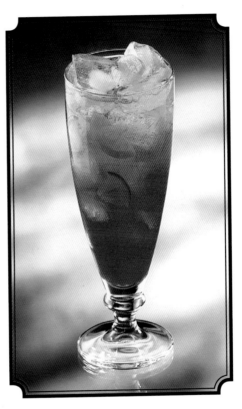

Serves 1

—

Ingredients

2 ounces grenadine

2 ounces fresh lemon
or lime juice

lemonade

fresh lemon or lime slices,
to garnish

1. Pour the grenadine and citrus juice into an ice-filled highball glass.

2. Top with lemonade and finish with slices of lemon or lime.

DUSTY SUNRISE

Serves 1

Ingredients

3 ounces orange juice

1½ ounces lemon juice

1½ ounces grenadine

sparkling water

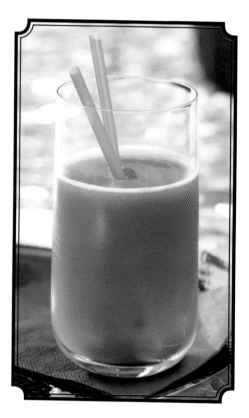

1. Fill a chilled tall glass halfway with ice and pour the orange juice, lemon juice, and grenadine over it.

2. Stir together well and top with sparkling water.

JUICY JULEP

Serves 1

—

Ingredients

1½ ounces orange juice

1½ ounces pineapple juice

1½ ounces lime juice

¾ ounce raspberry syrup

4 crushed fresh mint leaves

ginger ale

fresh mint sprig, to garnish

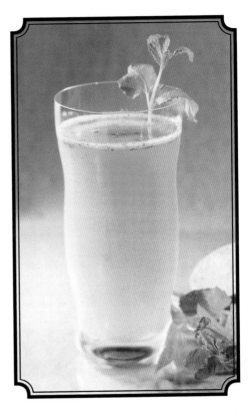

1. Shake the first five ingredients vigorously over ice until well frosted.

2. Strain into a chilled Collins glass, top with ginger ale and stir gently. Garnish with mint sprig.

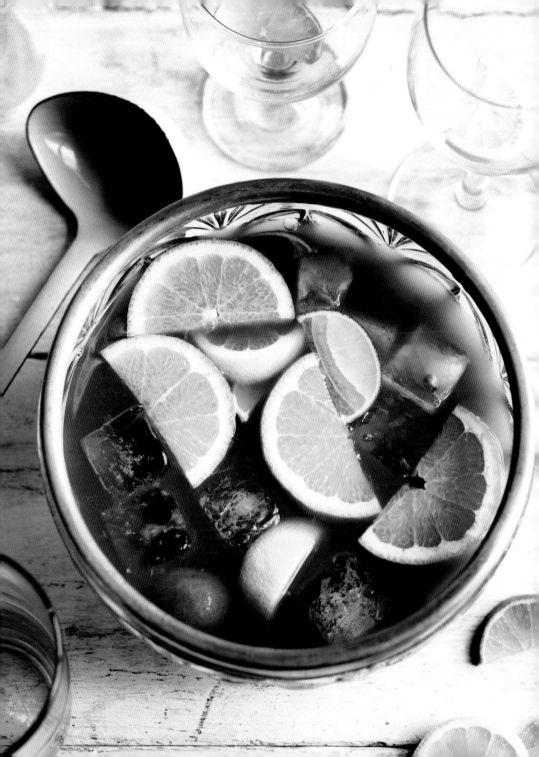

SOFT SANGRIA

Serves 10

Ingredients

40 ounces grape juice, chilled

10 ounces orange juice, chilled

2½ ounces cranberry juice, chilled

2 ounces lemon juice

2 ounces lime juice

3½ ounces simple syrup

lemon, orange, and lime slices, to garnish

1. Put the grape juice, orange juice, cranberry juice, lemon juice, lime juice, and simple syrup into a chilled punch bowl and stir well.

2. Add ice and garnish with the slices of lemon, orange, and lime.

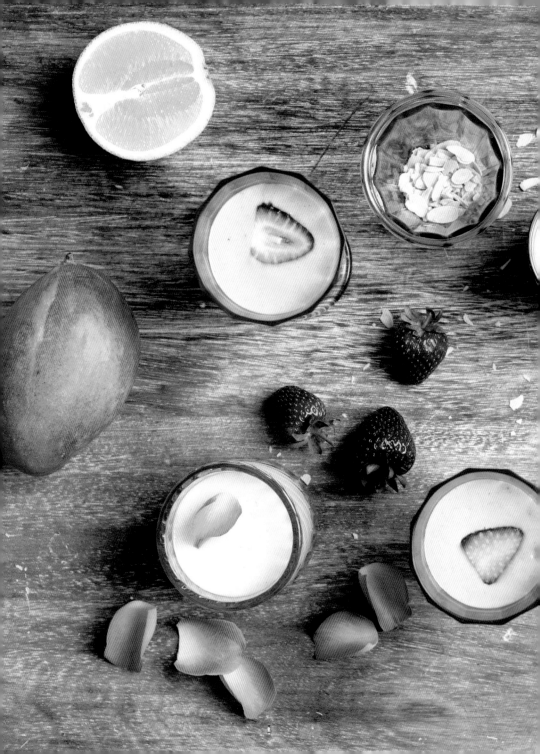

Chapter 3

CREAM

For a luscious mocktail experience we present dreamy drinks with a creamy inclination—from yogurt, cream, and ice cream to velvety mixtures of banana, nectarine, carrot juice, honey, coconut cream, and avocado.

AVOCADO THYME

Serves 1

Ingredients

½ large avocado

pinch of salt

2½ tablespoons fresh lime juice

2 teaspoons agave syrup

3 fresh thyme sprigs

2 ounces soda water

1. Mash the avocado with the salt in a cocktail shaker until smooth.

2. Add ice cubes, lime juice, agave syrup, and 2 thyme sprigs and shake hard.

3. Double strain into a hurricane glass and top with the soda water.

4. Garnish with the remaining thyme sprig.

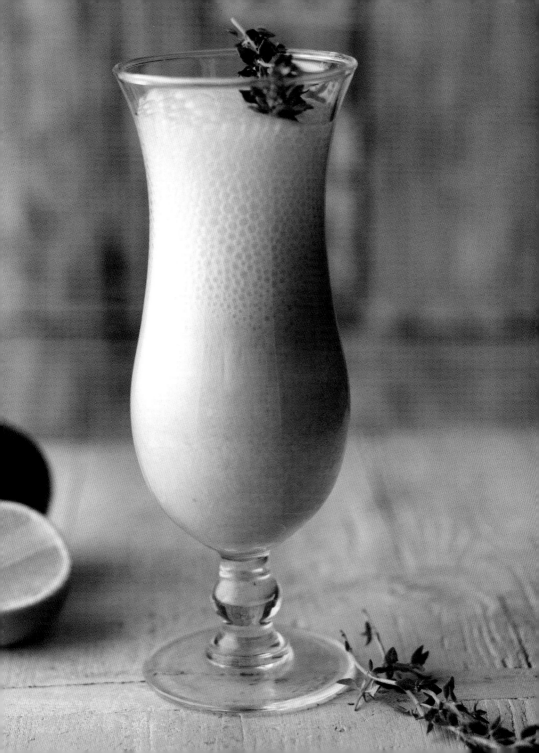

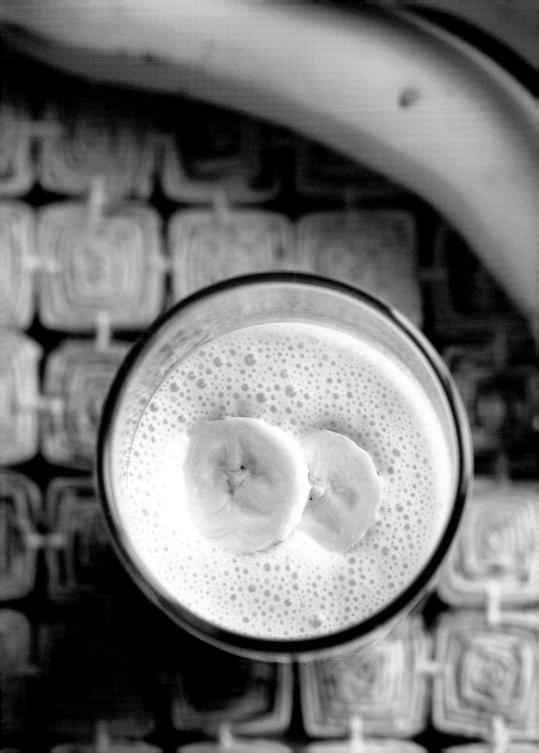

PEANUT CUP

Serves 1

Ingredients

2 tablespoons pureed banana

2 teaspoons peanut butter powder

5 ounces skim milk

banana slices, to garnish

1. Put all the ingredients into a cocktail shaker filled with ice cubes.

2. Shake hard and pour directly from the shaker into a highball glass.

3. Garnish with banana slices.

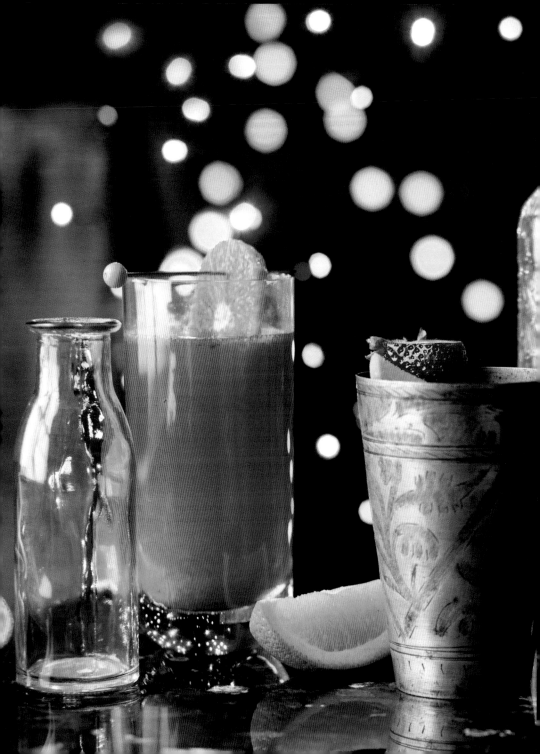

THE MOCKTAIL
GARNISH

Whether a bright piece of fruit, a briny olive, or a festive umbrella, the garnish has a solid place in the history of mixed drinks. In the case of fruit wedges, slices, or twists, the garnish imbues a flavor of juice or citrus oil to the drink. Likewise, an olive or onion lends a whisper of savory flavor. There are also bright red cherries, adding sweetness and color to drinks.

When cutting citrus wedges and slices, top and tail the fruit ends and cut the fruit in half lengthwise. For wedges, cut each side in half, and in half again, giving you eight wedges per fruit. For slices, slice each half to a width of ¼ inch. To create a citrus peel, use a vegetable peeler, fruit knife, or channel knife. Start by cutting the bottom off the fruit and cut away from you. Remove the pith before using.

Flamed orange is a dramatic garnish that will impart a burnt orange flavor to drinks. To do this, cut a thick piece of peel, hold it lengthwise between your thumb and forefinger and using a lighter, gently burn the outer skin of the peel to draw out the oils. Then squeeze the orange peel inward to express the oils through the flame. Care should be taken when attempting this technique.

Garnish skewers can be made from bamboo, wood, plastic, or even rosemary sprigs. Generally used for softer fruits such as berries, skewers can also create more intricate garnishes such as an apple fan. Sprigs of herbs are another garnish idea—these reflect the ingredients in the mocktail and endow the drink with a deeper aroma. Herb sprigs also have great natural panache!

AMANDINE

Serves 1

Ingredients

3 ounces peach juice

6 ounces cold milk

few drops almond extract

1–2 tablespoons clover honey

1 small egg

toasted almonds, to garnish

1. Shake the first five ingredients together until well frosted.

2. Pour into a large cocktail glass or wine glass and sprinkle the almonds on top.

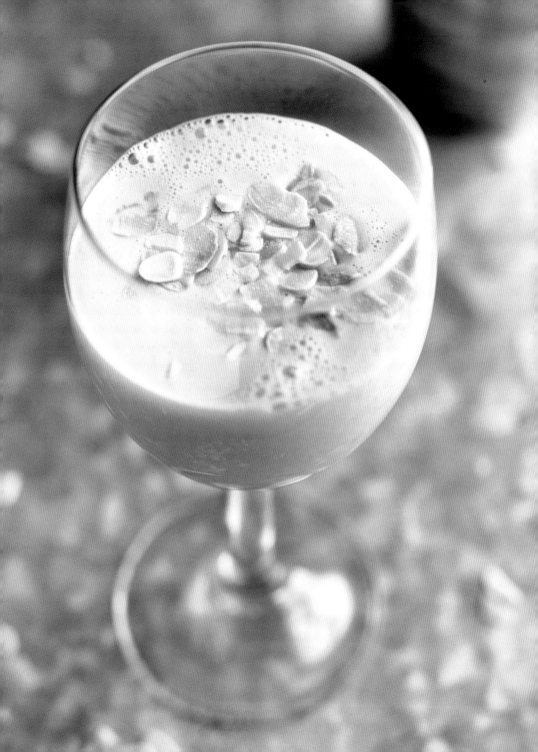

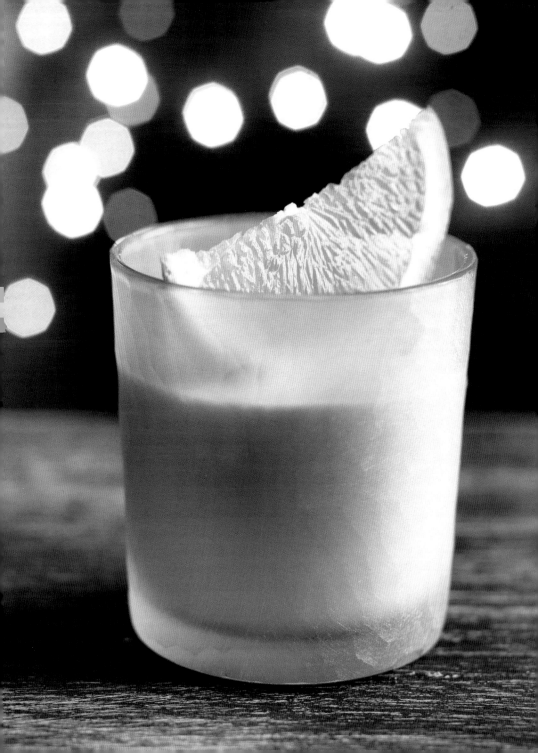

CARROT CREAM

Serves 1

Ingredients

3 ounces carrot juice

4¼ ounces light cream

3 ounces orange juice

1 egg yolk

orange slice, to garnish

1. Pour the carrot juice, cream, and orange juice over ice in a shaker and add the egg yolk. Shake vigorously until well mixed.

2. Strain into a chilled glass and garnish with the slice of orange.

MANGO LASSI

Serves 2

Ingredients

4 ounces plain yogurt

8 ounces milk

1 tablespoon rose water

3 tablespoons honey

1 ripe mango, peeled and diced

rose petals, to garnish

1. Pour the yogurt and milk into a blender and process until combined. Add the rose water and honey and process until blended, then add the mango and ice cubes and blend until smooth.

2. Pour into chilled glasses. Garnish with rose petals.

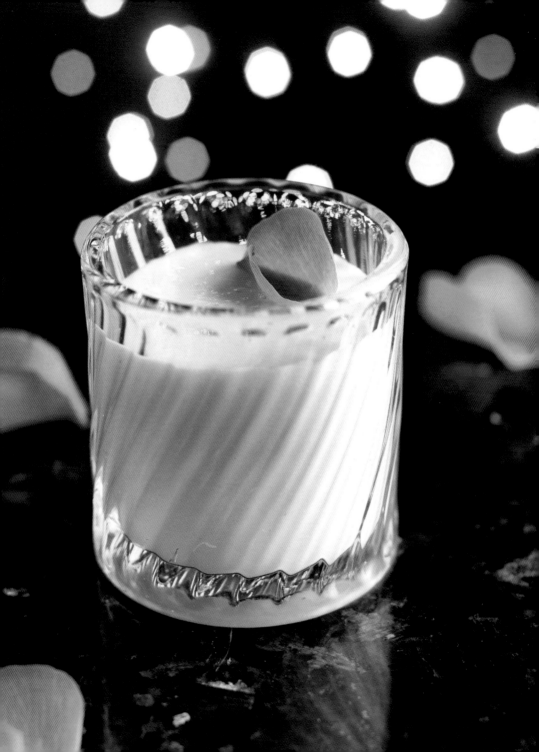

MINI COLADA

Serves 2

—

Ingredients

9 ounces milk

4½ ounces coconut cream

9 ounces pineapple juice

To Garnish

2 pineapple chunks

2 pineapple leaves

2 maraschino cherries

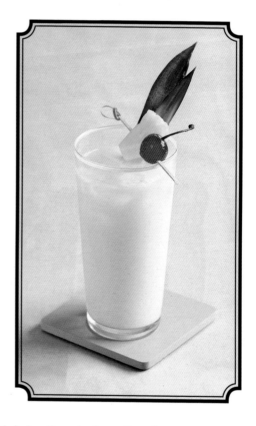

1. Put 4–6 ice cubes into a cocktail shaker. Pour in the milk and coconut cream.

3. Add the pineapple juice and shake vigorously until well frosted.

4. Fill 2 highball glasses halfway with ice, strain the liquid into them, and garnish with the pineapple chunk, pineapple leaf, and cherry.

COCO BERRY

Serves 1

Ingredients

3¼ ounces raspberries

1½ ounces coconut cream

5 ounces pineapple juice

pineapple wedge, to garnish

a few raspberries, to garnish

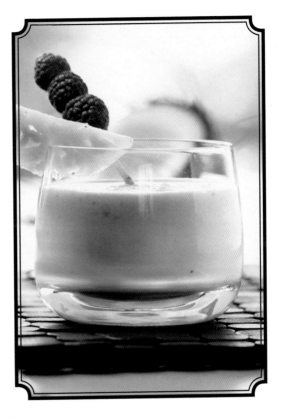

1. Press the raspberries through a strainer with the back of a spoon and transfer the puree to a blender.

2. Add the crushed ice, coconut cream, and pineapple juice and blend until smooth, then pour the mixture, without straining, into a chilled lowball glass.

3. Garnish with a pineapple wedge and fresh raspberries.

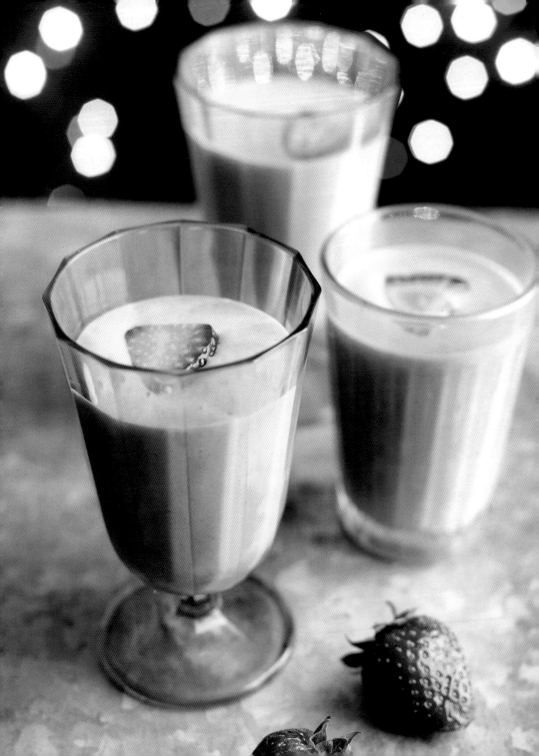

BABYLOVE

Serves 2

Ingredients

10 ounces milk

12–14 strawberries, hulled

½ ripe avocado

1½ ounces lemon juice

1. Place all the ingredients except 2 strawberries in a blender and blend for 15–20 seconds, until smooth.

2. Pour into iced tall glasses and garnish each glass with slices of strawberry.

BEE POLLEN & NECTARINE SHAKE

Serves 2

—

Ingredients

2 ripe nectarines, quartered

7 ounces 2% milk

2 tablespoons Greek yogurt

1 tablespoon bee pollen

1 teaspoon honey

1 teaspoon bee
pollen, to garnish

2 slices nectarine, to garnish

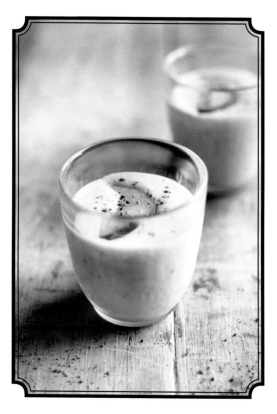

1. Place the the nectarines, milk, yogurt, bee pollen, and honey in a blender and blend until smooth. Add the ice cubes and blend again until completely combined.

2. Pour the milkshake into chilled glasses and garnish with the bee pollen and a fresh slice of nectarine.

MOCHA SLUSH

Serves 1

—

Ingredients

3½ ounces coffee syrup

1½ ounces chocolate syrup

7 ounces milk

grated chocolate, to garnish

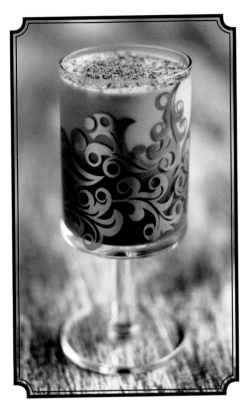

1. Add 4–6 ice cubes to a blender with the coffee and chocolate syrups and milk. Blend until slushy.

2. Pour into a chilled glass and sprinkle with grated chocolate.

FRUIT COOLER

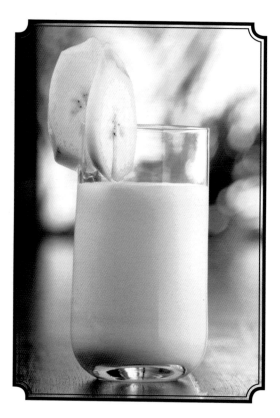

Serves 2

—

Ingredients

8 ounces orange juice

4 ounces plain yogurt

2 eggs

2 bananas, sliced and frozen

fresh banana slices,
to garnish

1. Pour the orange juice and yogurt into a food processor and process gently until combined.

2. Add the eggs and frozen bananas and process until smooth.

3. Pour the mixture into highball or hurricane glasses and garnish the rims with slices of fresh banana.

APPLE PIE CREAM

Serves 1

—

Ingredients

6 ounces apple juice

1 small scoop vanilla
ice cream

soda water

cinnamon sugar, to garnish

apple slice, to garnish

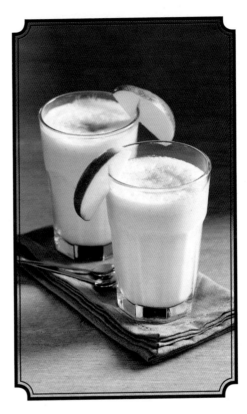

1. Put 4–6 ice cubes into a blender then add the apple juice and ice cream.

2. Blend for 10–15 seconds until frothy and frosted.
Pour into a glass and top with soda water.

3. Sprinkle the cinnamon sugar on top and garnish with an apple slice.

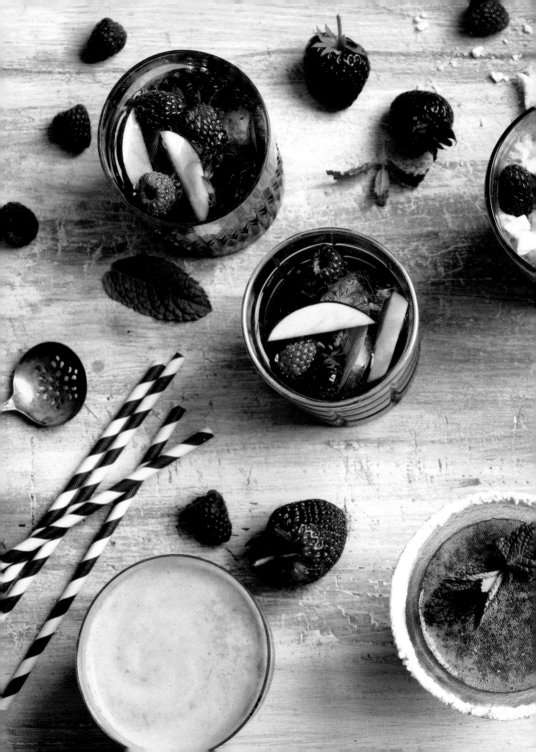

Chapter 4

BERRY

Berries are bountiful in nature and in this collection of mocktails. Presented in solo glory or in lively berry mixes, delight in them all—blackberries, juniper berries, strawberries, raspberries, grapes, and cranberries.

BLACKBERRY COLLINS

Serves 1

Ingredients

9 fresh blackberries

3 teaspoons blood orange juice

4 ounces sparkling water

blood orange slice, to garnish

Lemonade Syrup

4 lemons

½ cup sugar

5 ounces water

1. To make the lemonade syrup, zest and juice the lemons. Add to a saucepan with the sugar and water. Place over medium head until the sugar has dissolved.

2. Strain the mixture and leave to cool. Then pour into a clean bottle and store in the refrigerator for up to 4 weeks.

3. Muddle 8 of the blackberries in a cocktail shaker with the orange juice.

4. Strain into a highball glass and top with the lemonade syrup and sparkling water.

5. Garnish with the remaining blackberry and a blood orange slice.

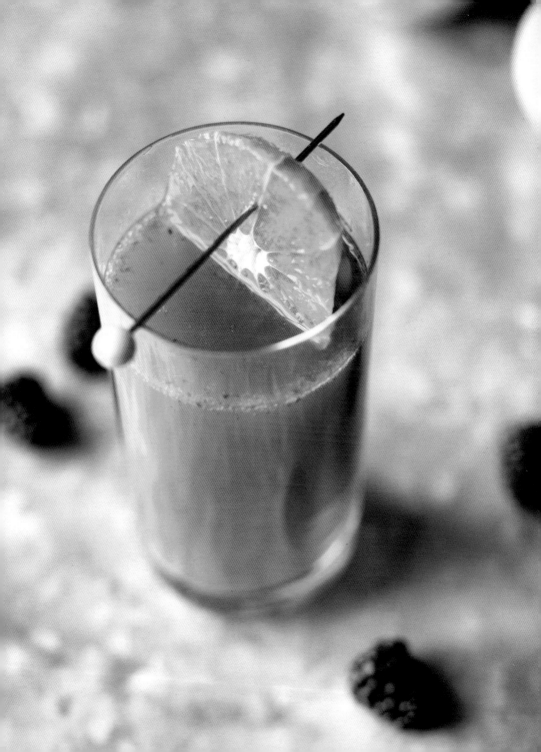

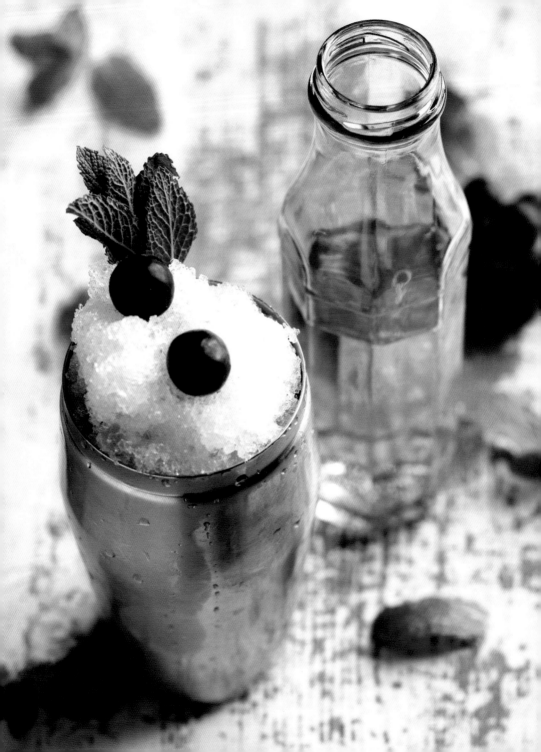

JUNIPER JULEP

Serves 1

Ingredients

17 ounces white grape juice

8–10 juniper berries

½ teaspoon agave syrup

2 teaspoons fresh lime juice

5 fresh fresh mint leaves

fresh mint sprig, to garnish

2 juniper berries, to garnish

1. Pour the grape juice into a pitcher. Add the juniper berries, stir well, then leave to infuse for 3 hours. Strain the juice into a clean bottle and store in the refrigerator for up to one month.

2. Mix the agave syrup and lime juice in a julep tin or highball glass to dissolve the syrup.

3. Bruise the mint leaves and add to the tin.

4. Fill the tin with crushed ice, then pour in 4 ounces of the infused grape juice. Stir the mixture through the ice.

5. Top with more crushed ice, garnish with a mint sprig, and two juniper berries.

STRAWBERRY MULE

Serves 1

—

Ingredients

3 fresh strawberries

2 ounces pineapple juice

2 teaspoons fresh lime juice

3½ ounces ginger beer

½ strawberry, to garnish

lime wedge, to garnish

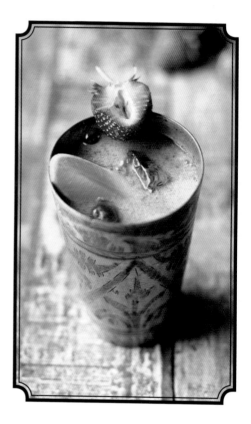

1. Muddle the strawberries in a copper mule mug or a highball glass.

2. Add the pineapple juice and lime and stir well to mix.

3. Add ice cubes to fill the mug. Top with the ginger beer and stir again.

4. Garnish with a strawberry half and a lime wedge.

SUPER BERRY HI-BALL

Serves 1

—

Ingredients

4 strawberries

6 raspberries

2 teaspoons fresh lime juice

2 fresh basil leaves

1 teaspoon agave syrup

soda water

berry skewer, to garnish

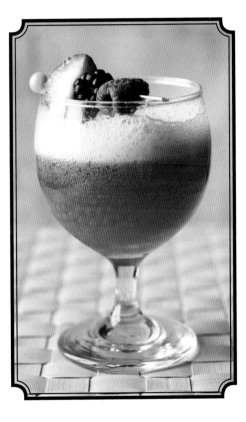

1. Muddle the strawberries, raspberries, lime juice, basil, and agave syrup in a cocktail shaker.

2. Fill the shaker with ice cubes and shake hard.

3. Fill a large wine glass with ice cubes and strain the liquid into the glass.

4. Top with soda water and stir gently. Garnish with a berry skewer.

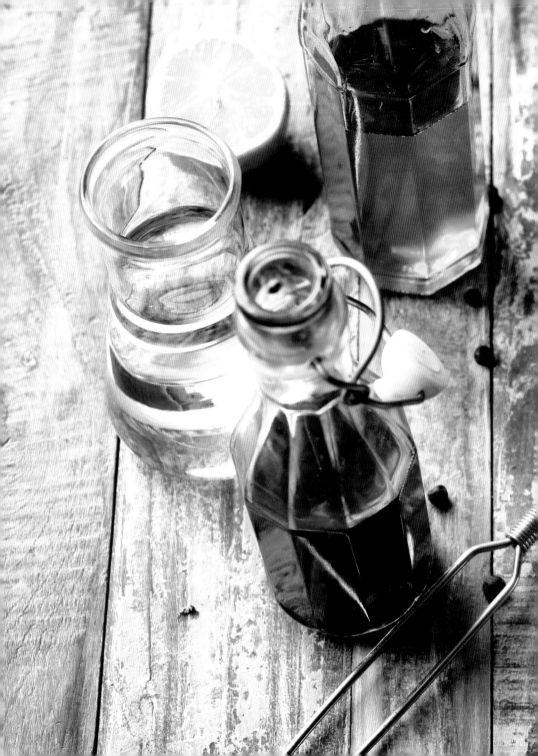

MAKING A
SYRUP

A syrup—a combination of sugar and water—will sweeten and add flavor to mocktails and cocktails. There are two ways to make homemade syrups, a hot process and a cold process. Using the hot method is quicker and can give a more mellow flavor syrup, whereas one made with a cold process provides a more vibrant flavor, and generally one that is truer to the original ingredients. The following recipe is made using the cold process. This syrup works wonderfully topped with light tonic water or soda water. It can also be shaken with apple juice and fresh mint for a mocktail twist on a julep.

BASIL & LIME SYRUP

peels from 3 limes
1 ounce fresh basil leaves;
1¾ cups superfine sugar
7 ounces cold water

1. Muddle the lime peels, basil leaves, and sugar together in a bowl. Cover the bowl in plastic wrap and set aside for at least 2 hours.

2. Remove the peels from the sugar and add the water. Place the contents in a sealed container and shake hard to dissolve the sugar.

3. Pour the mixture through a fine-mesh strainer and decant into a clean, clip-top bottle. This syrup will store in the refrigerator for up to 4 weeks.

CRANBERRY PUNCH

Serves 10

Ingredients

48 ounces cranberry juice

15 ounces water

1½ teaspoons ground ginger

¾ teaspoon cinnamon

¾ teaspoon freshly
grated nutmeg

frozen cranberries and
their leaves, to garnish

1. Put the first five ingredients into a saucepan and bring to a boil. Reduce the heat and simmer for 5 minutes.

2. Remove from the heat and pour into a heatproof pitcher or bowl. Chill in the refrigerator.

3. Remove from the refrigerator, put ice into the serving glasses, pour in the punch, and garnish with cranberries and their leaves on cocktail sticks.

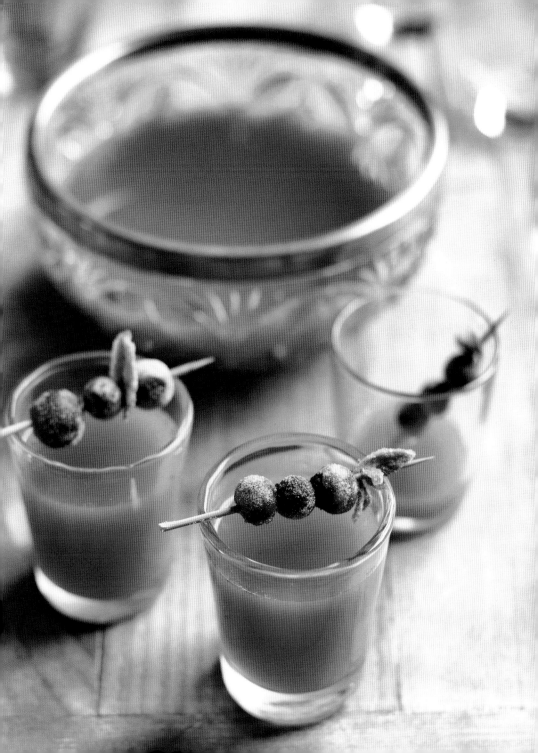

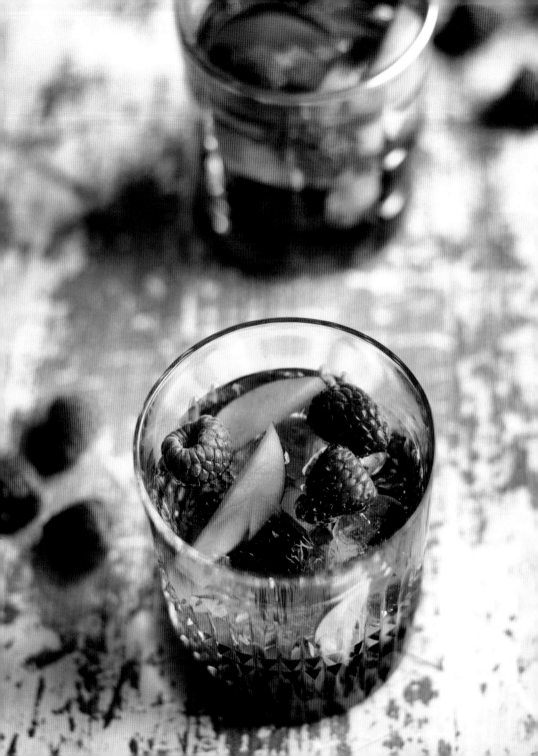

RASPBERRY COOLER

Serves 2

Ingredients

2 teaspoons raspberry syrup

16 ounces chilled apple juice

fresh raspberries, to garnish

apple pieces, to garnish

1. Add ice and 1 teaspoon of raspberry syrup to each glass.

2. Fill each glass with 8 ounces of apple juice and stir well.

3. Garnish with the raspberries and pieces of apple.

CRANBERRY ENERGIZER

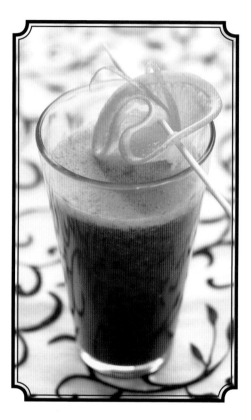

Serves 2

—

Ingredients

10 ounces cranberry juice

4 ounces orange juice

2 ounces fresh raspberries

1 tablespoon lemon juice

fresh orange slices,
to garnish

1. Pour the cranberry juice and orange juice into a blender and blend gently until combined.

2. Add the raspberries and lemon juice and blend until smooth.

3. Strain into glasses and garnish with the slices of orange.

BERRY BERRY RED

Serves 2

—

Ingredients

2 ounces raspberries

6 ounces cranberry juice

6 ounces raspberry juice

1 small meringue, crumbled

blackberry-flavored
sparkling water

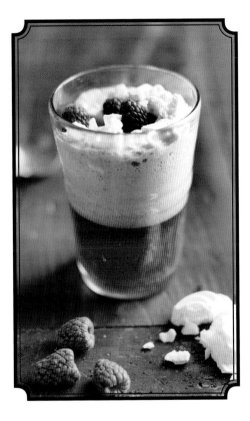

1. Set aside a couple of raspberries for later. In a blender, blend the rest of the fruit with the juices and crushed ice.

2. Divide the fruit slush between two tall glasses and top with the sparkling water.

3. Garnish with raspberries and the crumbled meringue.

FAUX KIR ROYALE

Serves 1

Ingredients

2¼ ounces raspberry syrup

sparkling apple juice, chilled

1. Put 4–6 ice cubes into a mixing glass. Then pour in the raspberry syrup.

2. Stir well to mix and strain into a chilled wine glass.

3. Top up with sparkling apple juice and stir.

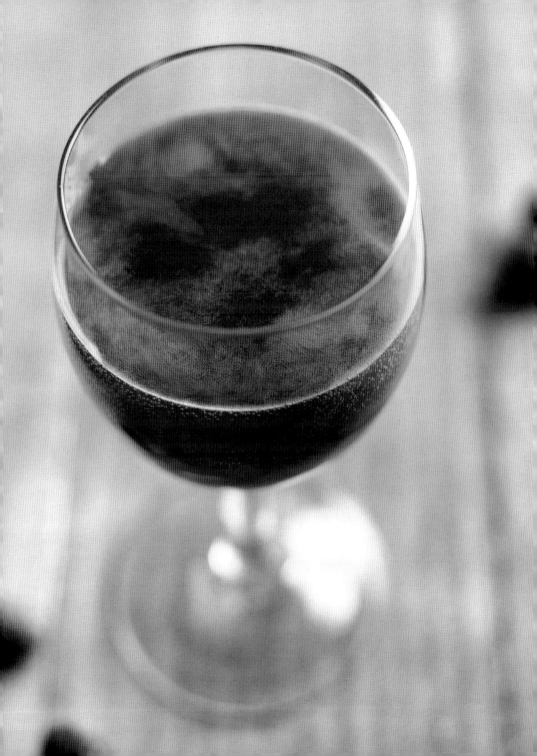

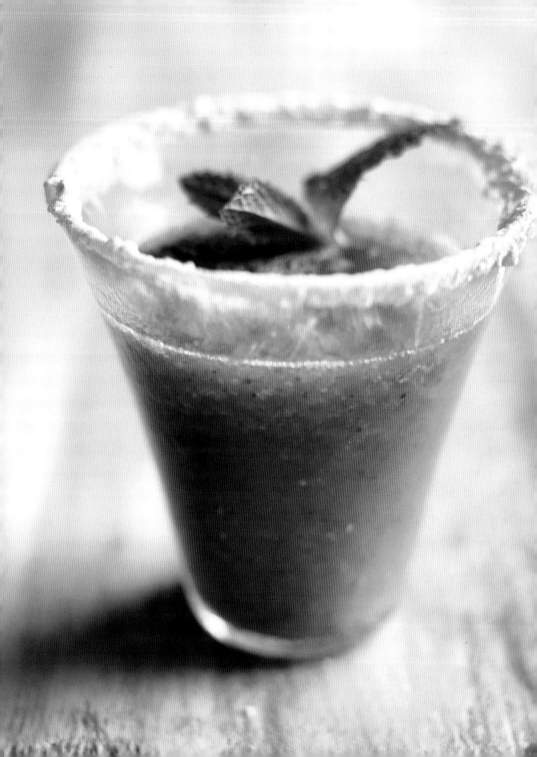

STRAWBERRY CRUSH

Serves 1

Ingredients

1 lemon wedge

1 teaspoon confectioners' sugar

2 ounces ripe strawberries

juice of ½ lemon

5 ounces lemonade, chilled

sugar, to taste

fresh mint sprig, to garnish

1. Place confectioners' sugar on a small plate. Run the lemon wedge around the rim of the glass, then dip in the confectioners' sugar. Leave to dry.

2. Hull the strawberries and blend with the lemon juice, lemonade, crushed ice, and sugar for 2–3 minutes, until smooth but frothy.

3. Pour into the sugared glass and garnish with mint.

SPARKLING PEACH MELBA

Serves 1

Ingredients

2 ounces raspberries, pureed

6 ounces peach juice

sparkling water

1. Shake the raspberry puree and peach juice over ice vigorously until well frosted.

2. Strain into a chilled tumbler, top with sparkling water, and stir gently.

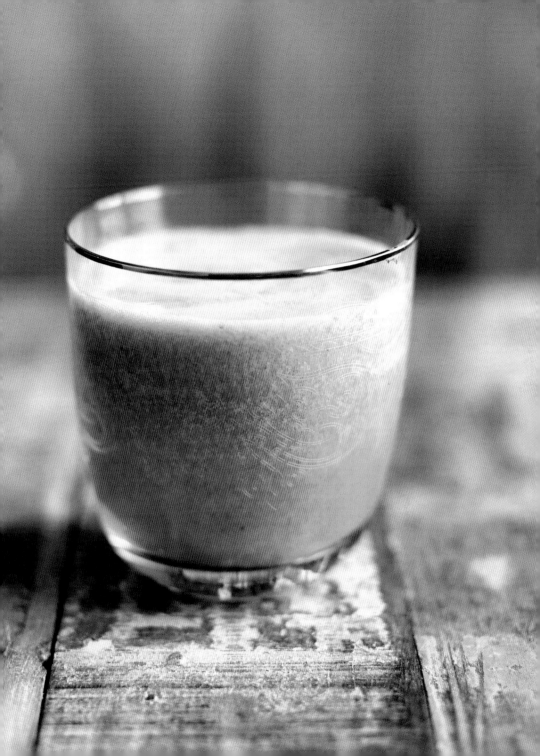

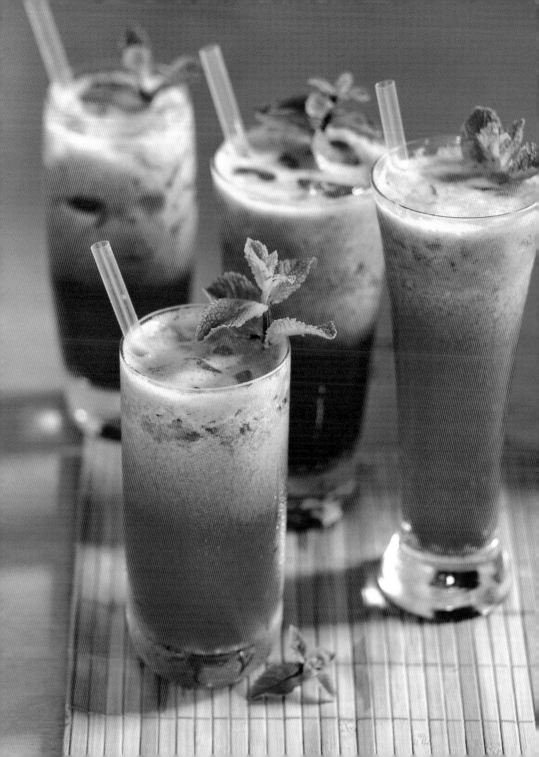

VIRGIN RASPBERRY COOLERS

Serves 4

Ingredients

2 lemons

1 cup confectioners' sugar

4 ounces raspberries

4 drops vanilla extract

sparkling water

fresh mint sprigs, to garnish

1. Cut the ends off the lemons, then scoop out and chop the flesh.

2. Put the lemon flesh in a blender with the sugar, raspberries, vanilla extract, and 4–6 ice cubes. Blend for 2–3 minutes.

3. Half-fill four highball glasses with ice and strain in the lemon mixture.

4. Top with sparkling water and garnish with the mint sprigs.

MEMORY LANE

Serves 1

Ingredients

10 blackberries

1 tablespoon confectioners' sugar

juice of ½ lemon

juice of ½ lime

lemonade

1. Reserve a few berries. Place the remaining fruit in a chilled tumbler with the sugar and crush until well mashed.

2. Add the fruit juices and a few ice cubes, then top with lemonade. Garnish with the reserved whole berries.

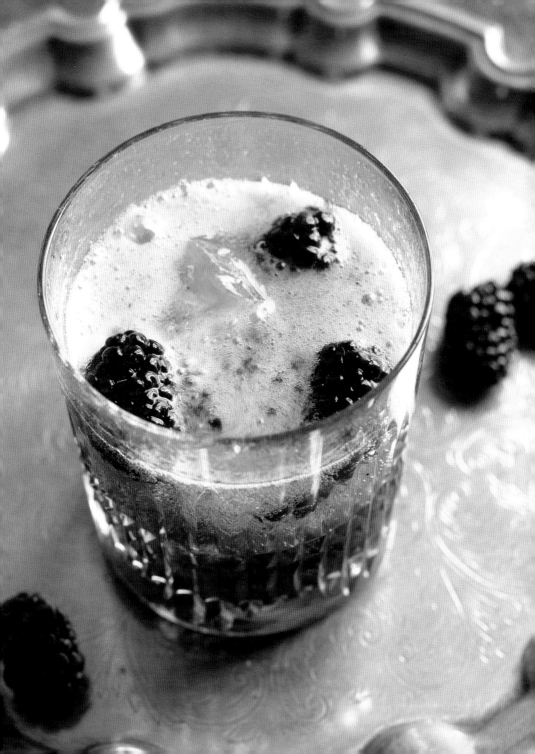

CRANBERRY & ORANGE CRUSH

Serves 2

—

Ingredients

juice of 2 blood oranges

5 ounces cranberry juice

2 tablespoons raspberry
or other fruit syrup

raspberries, to garnish

sugar, to taste

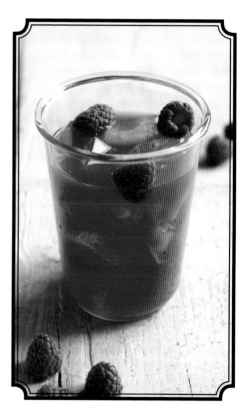

1. Shake the first three ingredients with ice together.

2. Pour straight into a tall ice-filled glass. Garnish with raspberries. Serve immediately.
This is a long and refreshing drink, but it can be sharp, so taste first, then sweeten if necessary

CHERRY ORCHARD

Serves 1

Ingredients

1½ ounces apple juice

1½ ounces pear juice

3 ounces cranberry juice

pink lemonade or cherryade

fresh or maraschino
cherries, to garnish

pineapple wedge, to garnish

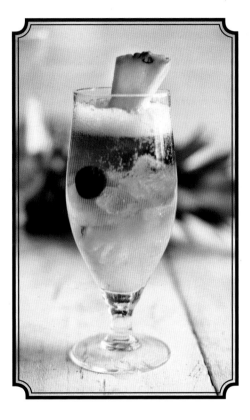

1. Mix the fruit juices together over ice in a chilled glass.

2. Fill with lemonade to taste and garnish with cherries and pineapple.

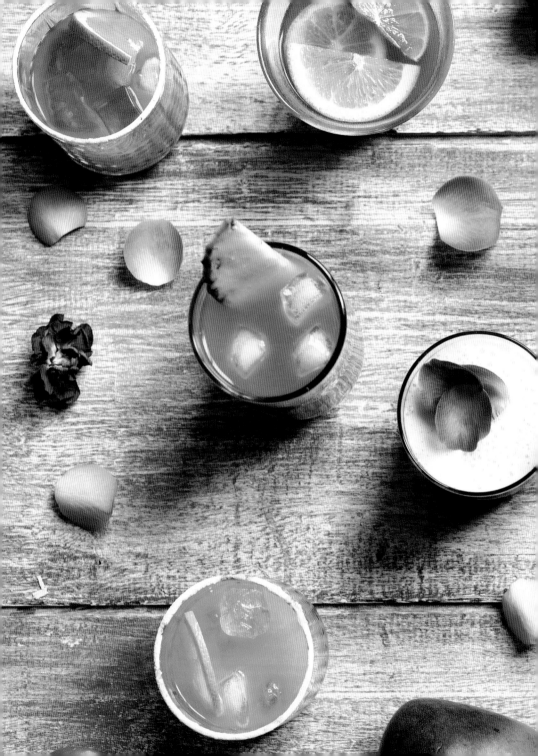

Chapter 5

TROPIC

In search of some soft-drink sunshine? Overflowing with exotic, tropical ingredients, these mocktails feature mango, melon, kiwi, passion fruit, guava, and pineapple, and carry a guaranteed feel-good factor.

COCO KIWI KIWI

Serves 1

Ingredients

2 teaspoons pineapple juice

2 tablespoons coconut water

3½ ounces ginger ale

2 kiwi slices, to garnish

pineapple leaf, to garnish

Kiwi Shrub

15 kiwis, peeled and quartered

1¾ cups sugar

12 ounces cider vinegar

1. To make the kiwi shrub, add the kiwi fruit to a bowl with the sugar, and mix well. Cover and chill in the refrigerator for 1 hour.

2. Muddle the mixture, re-cover and leave in the refrigerator overnight.

3. Strain the mixture and add the vinegar, then shake well and leave in the refrigerator overnight. Strain through a cheese cloth or fine sieve and store in the refrigerator in a clean jar for up to one week.

4. Put 2 tablespoons of the kiwi shrub into a cocktail shaker with the pineapple juice, coconut water, and ice cubes.

5. Strain into a highball glass filled with ice cubes. Top with the ginger ale and gently stir.

6. Garnish with kiwi slices and a pineapple leaf.

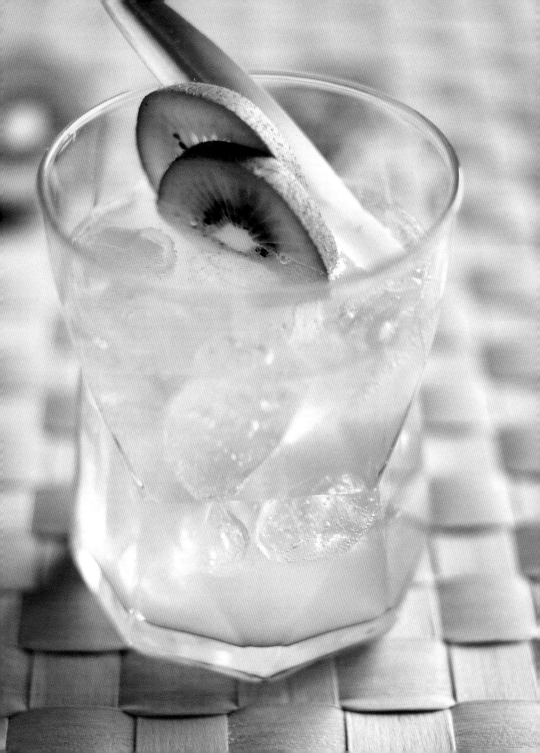

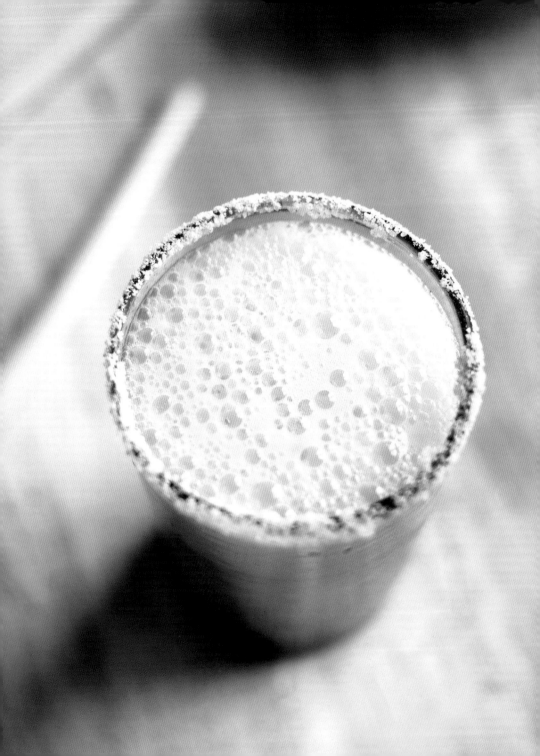

LEMONGRASS LAGERITA

Serves 1

Ingredients

juice of ½ lime

1 teaspoon salt

¼ lemongrass stalk, chopped

2 tablespoons mango juice

7 ounces nonalcoholic
lager, chilled

1. Dip a highball glass in
the lime juice and then in
the salt to give a salted rim.

2. Muddle the lemongrass with
the mango juice in a shaker
and strain into the glass.

3. Top with the lager.

MELON BELLINI

Serves 1

Ingredients

2 ounces pureed watermelon

½ teaspoon agave syrup

2 teaspoons apple juice

2 ounces ginger ale

thin watermelon slice, to garnish

1. Fill a cocktail shaker with ice cubes, add the watermelon puree, agave syrup, and apple juice and shake vigorously.

2. Strain into a chilled champagne flute and top with ginger ale.

3. Garnish with a watermelon slice.

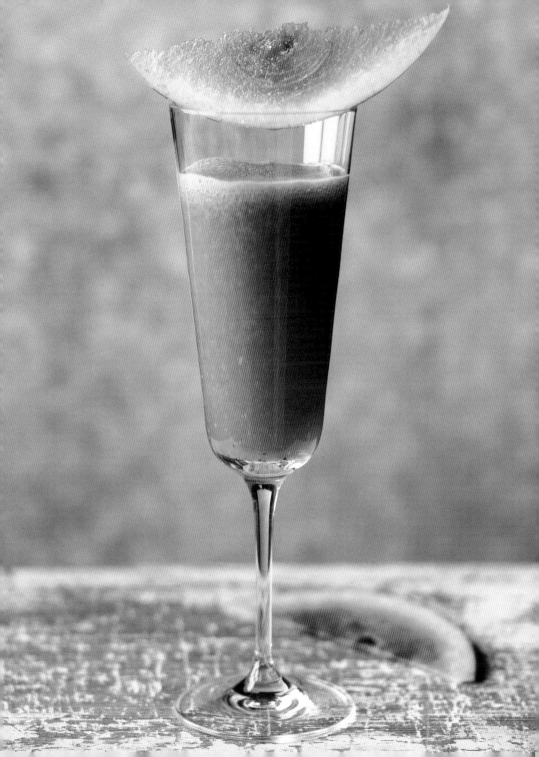

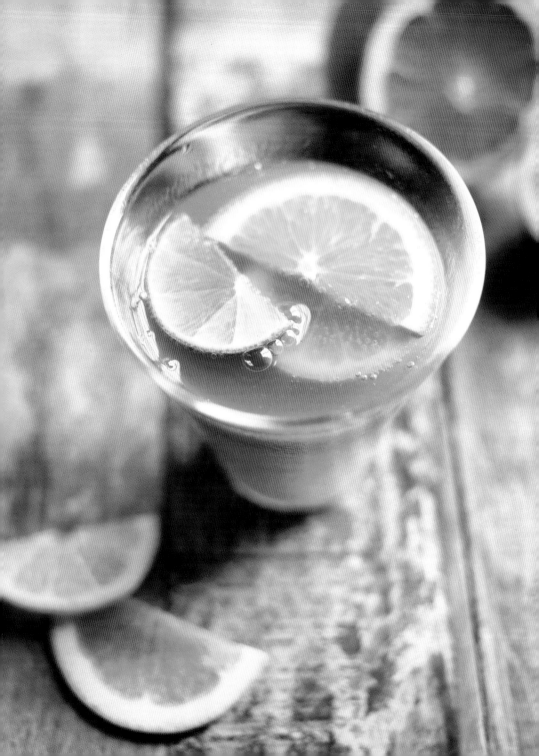

PINEAPPLE PIZAZZ

Serves 1

Ingredients

juice of ½ orange

juice of 1 lime

5 ounces pineapple juice

4–5 drops nonalcoholic
aromatic bitters

soda water or dry
ginger ale, to taste

fruit slices, to garnish

1. Shake the first
four ingredients well
together with ice.

2. Strain into a chilled glass
and fill with soda water to taste.

3. Finish with a few more
drops of bitters to taste,
garnish with slices of fruit.

ISLAND FRUIT COCKTAIL

Serves 1

Ingredients

1½ ounces pineapple juice

1½ ounces orange juice

¾ ounce lime juice

1½ ounces passion fruit juice

3 ounces guava juice

flower, to garnish

1. Shake all the juices together with crushed ice.

2. Strain into a chilled tall glass and garnish with a flower.

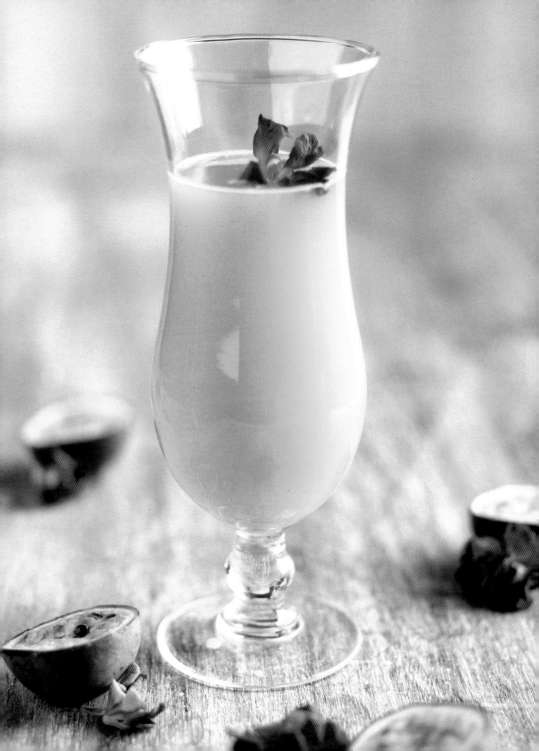

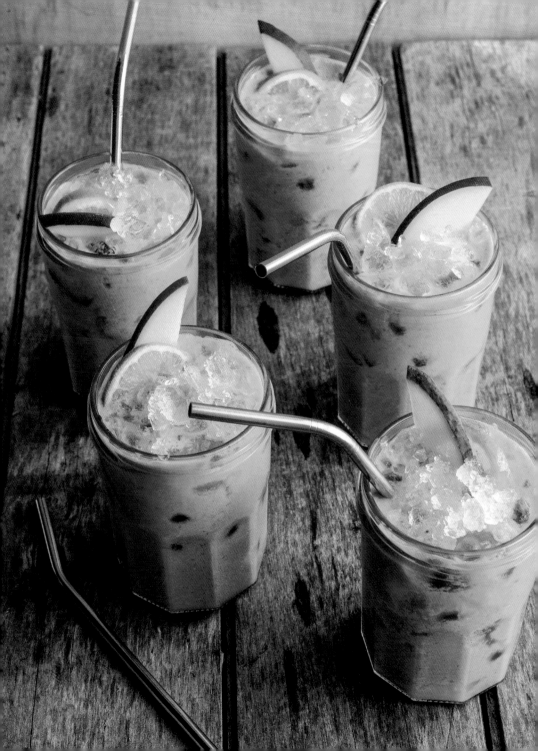

MELON & COCONUT MOCK MOJITO

Serves 1

Ingredients

¾ ounce spinach

1¾ ounces coconut flesh

7 ounces chilled water

3½ ounces cantaloupe melon,
peeled, deseeded, and chopped

1 tablespoon chopped fresh mint

juice of ½ lime

1¾ ounces mango, peeled,
stoned, and chopped, plus
1 extra slice to garnish

1. Place the spinach, coconut, and water in a blender and blend until smooth.

2. Add the melon, mint, lime juice, and mango, and blend until smooth and creamy.

3. Pour over crushed ice and serve immediately, garnished with a mango slice.

ISLAND COOLER

Serves 1

Ingredients

3 ounces orange juice

1½ ounces lemon juice

1½ ounces pineapple juice

1½ ounces papaya juice

½ teaspoon grenadine

sparkling water

pineapple wedges, to garnish

maraschino cherries, to garnish

1. Shake the fruit juices and grenadine vigorously over ice until well frosted.

2. Fill a Collins glass halfway with ice and pour in the cocktail.

3. Top with sparkling water and stir gently. Garnish with pineapple wedges and maraschino cherries.

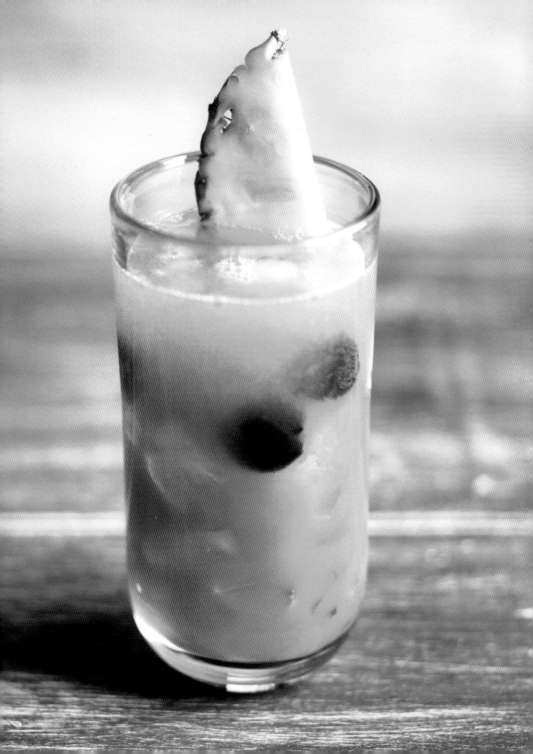

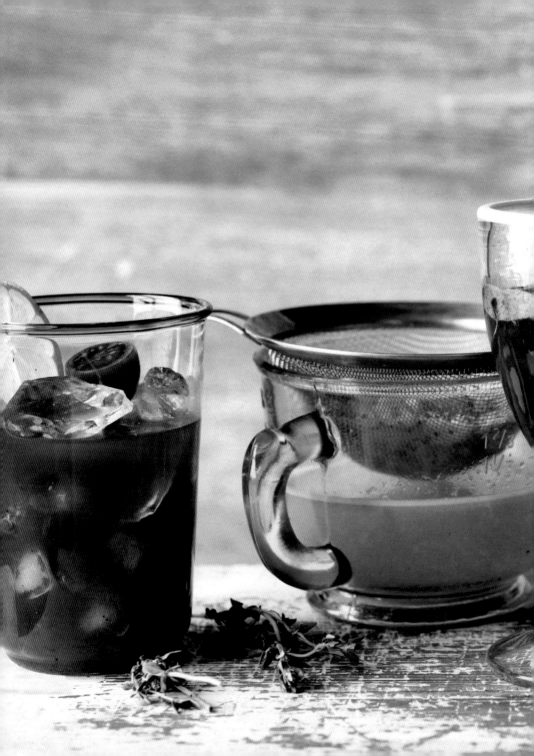

MAKING A
SHRUB

Shrubs provide both sweet and tart flavors and give depth to mocktails and cocktails. They can be made using a hot or a cold process. The cold process takes a little longer, but creates a purer and brighter fruit flavor. This fruit shrub, made with the cold process, is delicious topped with light tonic water, or with hot water and fresh ginger for a cold-busting beverage in the winter months.

STRAWBERRY & MIXED PEPPERCORN SHRUB

2 whole lemons, peeled
1½ ounces superfine sugar
23 ounces strawberries, hulled and quartered
1 teaspoon mixed peppercorns
7 ounces cider vinegar
1¾ ounces balsamic vinegar

1. Muddle the lemon peels and sugar together in a bowl. Cover the bowl with plastic wrap and set aside for at least an hour.

2. Remove the peels and add the strawberries and the mixed peppercorns to the sugar. Stir the ingredients to combine. Cover the bowl with plastic wrap again and place in the refrigerator for a couple of hours.

3. Remove the bowl from the refrigerator and muddle the berries into the sugar to press out as much juice as possible. Add the vinegar and stir again to mix well. Cover and return to the refrigerator for 2–3 days.

4. Remove from the refrigerator, muddle the mixture again, and pour through a fine mesh strainer into a clean mason jar or clip-top bottle.

5. Store in the refrigerator for a week, to allow the flavors to blend; shake before using. This shrub can be stored for up to 6 months.

6. Mix with and sparkling lemonade for a refreshing mocktail.

ORANGE & LIME ICED TEA

Serves 2

—

Ingredients

11 ounces chilled fresh tea

4 ounces orange juice

4 tablespoons lime juice

1–2 tablespoons sugar

lime wedges

orange slices, to garnish

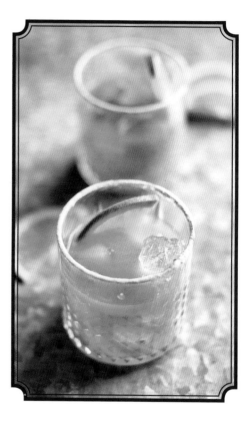

1. Add the orange juice, lime juice, and sugar to taste to the tea.

2. Take two glasses and rub the rims with a lime wedge,
then dip them in sugar to frost.

3. Fill the glasses with ice and pour in the tea.
Garnish with slices of orange.

BRIGHT GREEN COOLER

Serves 1

—

Ingredients

4½ ounces pineapple juice

3 ounces lime juice

1½ ounces green
peppermint syrup

ginger ale

cucumber strip, to garnish

lime slice, to garnish

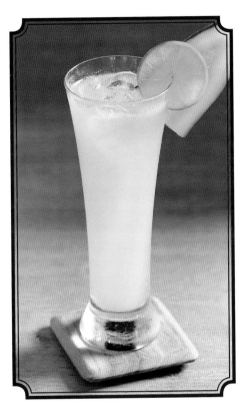

1. Put 4–6 ice cubes into a cocktail shaker.

2. Pour in the pineapple juice, lime juice, and peppermint
syrup and shake vigorously until well frosted.

3. Half-fill a highball glass with ice and strain the cocktail over it.

4. Top with ginger ale and garnish with the cucumber strip and lime slice.

TROPICAL COOLER

Serves 1

Ingredients

3 ounces passion fruit juice

3 ounces guava juice

3 ounces orange juice

1½ ounces coconut milk

1–2 teaspoon ginger syrup

slice of papaya, to garnish

1. Shake all the fruit juices with the coconut milk and ginger syrup vigorously over ice until well frosted.

2. Strain into a chilled highball glass or tall wine glass and garnish with a thin slice of papaya.

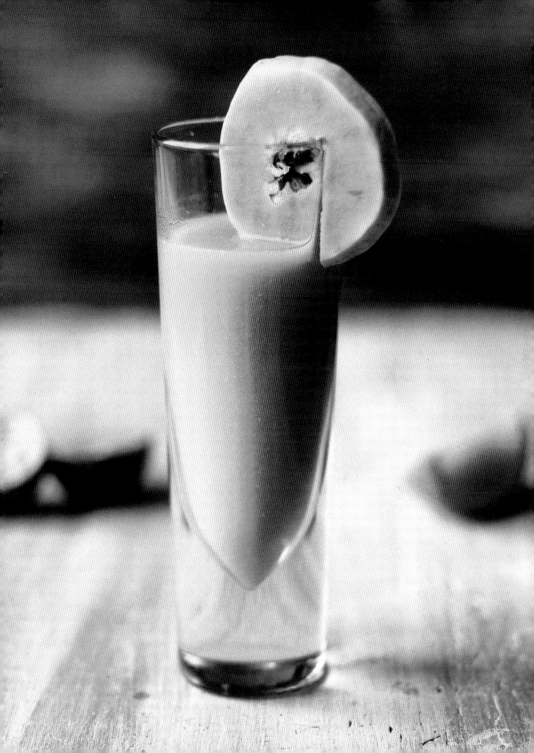

PASSIONATE FIZZ

Serves 1

—

Ingredients

½ ounce pomegranate juice

2 ounces fresh orange juice

1 ounce frozen passion
fruit pulp, thawed

¾ ounce simple syrup

sparkling water

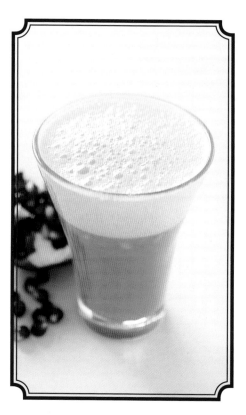

1. Add the first three ingredients to a blender with 3–4 ice cubes and blend until smooth.

2. Pour into a glass and top with sparkling water.

HEAVENLY DAYS

Serves 1

—

Ingredients

3 ounces hazelnut syrup

3 ounces lemon juice

1 teaspoon grenadine

sparkling water

slice of papaya, to garnish

1. Shake the syrup, lemon juice, and grenadine vigorously over ice until well frosted.

2. Fill a tumbler halfway with ice and strain the cocktail into the glass.

3. Top with sparkling water. Stir gently and garnish with a slice of papaya.

BABY BELLINI

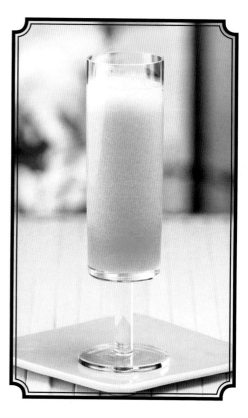

Serves 1

—

Ingredients

3 ounces peach juice

1½ ounces lemon juice

sparkling apple juice

1. Pour the peach juice and lemon juice into a chilled champagne flute and stir well.

2. Top with sparkling apple juice and stir again.

EYE OF THE HURRICANE

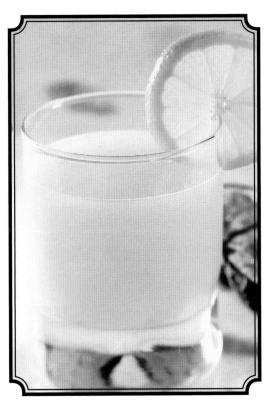

Serves 1

—

Ingredients

3 ounces passion fruit syrup

1½ ounces lime juice

bitter lemon

lemon slice, to garnish

1. Pour the passion fruit syrup and lime juice over ice in a mixing glass.

2. Stir well to mix and strain into a chilled tumbler.

3. Top with bitter lemon and dress with a slice of lemon.

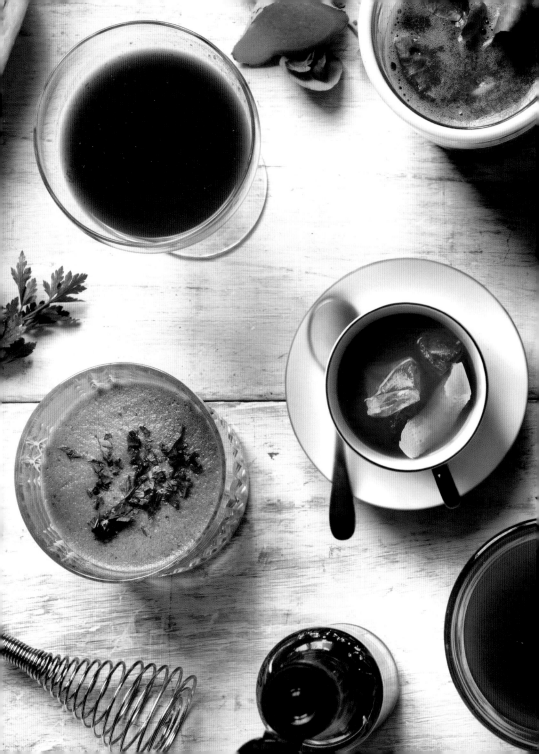

Chapter 6

KICK

Fancy some mixology spirit without the spirits? These mocktails have dynamic ingredients that make a bold mark—charred peppers, beets, espresso, matcha green tea, turmeric, hot pepper sauce, clam juice, and cayenne pepper.

BURNT ORANGE SOUR

Serves 1

Ingredients

6–8 Padrón or shishito peppers

17 ounces carrot juice

2 teaspoons fresh lemon juice

4 tablespoons fresh orange juice

charred pepper, to garnish

orange twist, to garnish

1. Use a chef's blowtorch to char the skins of the peppers.

2. Put the carrot juice in a pitcher. Leaving the charred skins on, add the peppers to the carrot juice, stir the contents, and leave to infuse for 1 hour.

3. Strain and pour the juice into a clean bottle and store in the refrigerator.

4. Fill a rocks glass with ice cubes. Add 3½ ounces of the infused carrot juice, lemon juice, and orange juice and stir.

5. Garnish with a charred pepper and an orange twist.

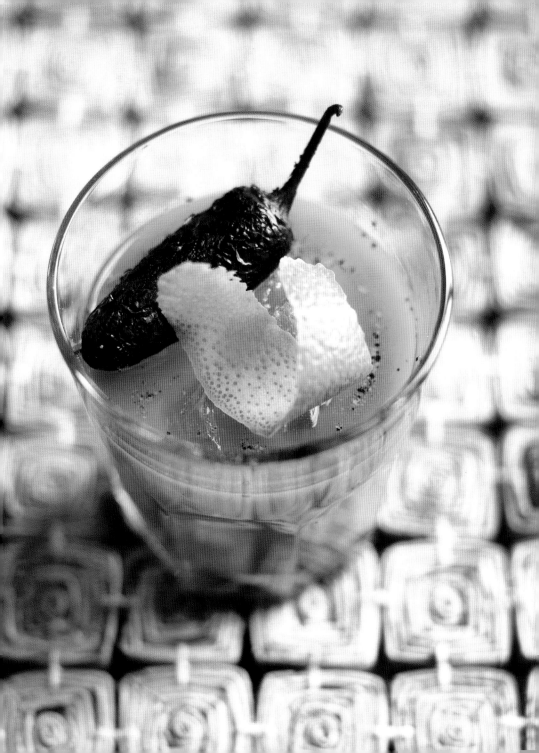

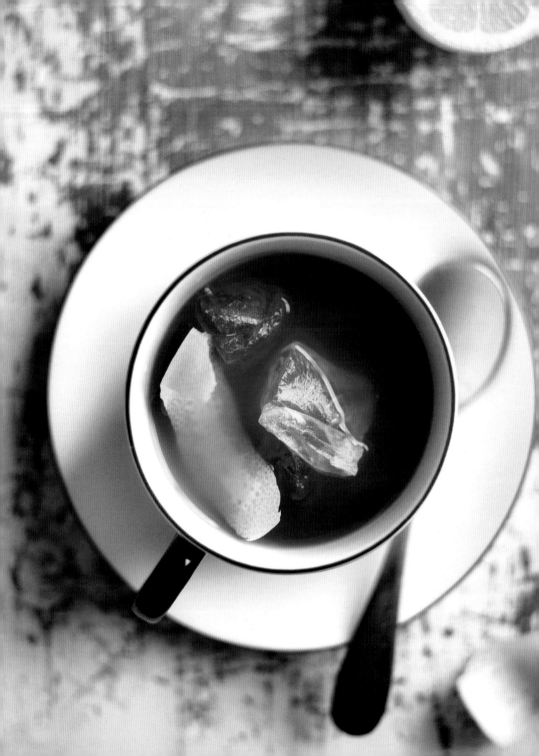

MATCHA COLLINS

Serves 1

Ingredients

2 slices fresh ginger

2 tablespoons fresh lemon juice

1 teaspoon honey

large pinch of matcha green tea powder

4 ounces ginger ale

lemon twist, to garnish

1. Whisk the matcha powder and honey into hot water.

2. Muddle the ginger with the lemon in a teacup. Add the tea mixture and stir well.

3. Add 4–5 ice cubes and slowly add the ginger ale.

4. Garnish with a lemon twist.

VIRGIN SMOKED MARY

Serves 1

Ingredients

2¾ ounces cold lapsang
souchong tea

3½ ounces tomato juice

2 teaspoons fresh lemon juice

3 dashes Worcestershire sauce

2 dashes hot pepper sauce

pinch of pepper

pinch of Himalayan pink salt

lemon wheel, to garnish

halved cherry tomato, to garnish

1. Add all ingredients except
garnishes into a tall glass
filled with ice cubes.

2. Stir well, garnish
with a lemon wheel
and a cherry tomato.

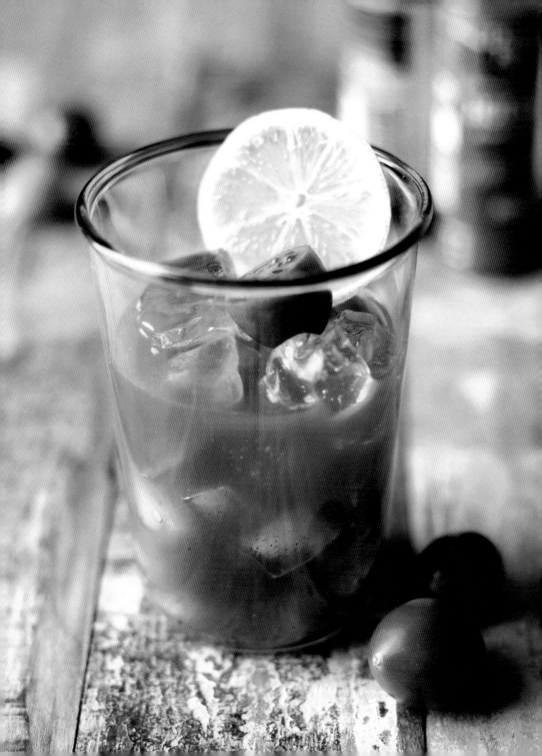

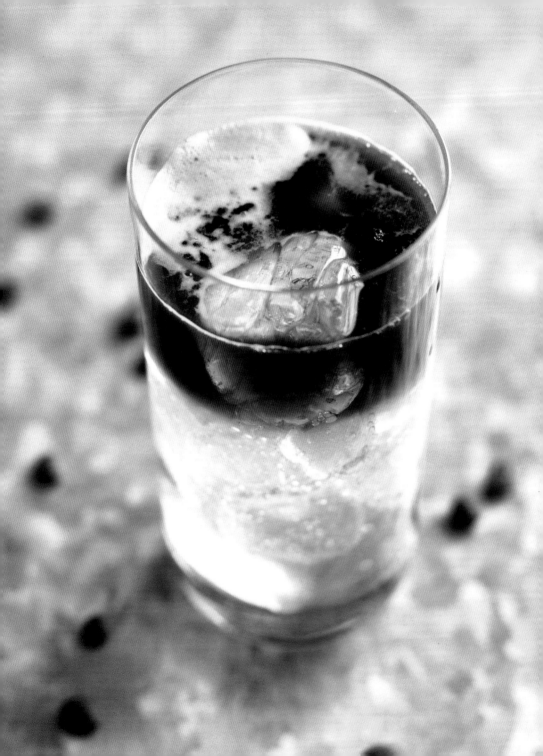

TURBO TONIC

Serves 1

Ingredients

7 ounces tonic water

2 tablespoons hot or
chilled espresso

Juniper Syrup

10–15 juniper berries

8½ ounces water

3 tablespoons sugar

1. To make the juniper syrup, add the juniper berries to a saucepan with the water and sugar and bring to the boil.

2. Remove from the heat and leave to cool, then strain into a clean bottle and store in the refrigerator.

3. Fill a highball glass with ice cubes. Add 2 teaspoons of the juniper syrup, pour over the tonic water and gently stir.

4. Place a spoon against the inside edge of the glass and slowly pour the espresso over the back of the spoon to float.

TURMERIC & TONIC

Serves 1

Ingredients

¼ teaspoon ground turmeric

7 ounces tonic water

2 teaspoons fresh lemon juice

lemon wheel, to garnish

1. Add ice cubes and turmeric to a highball glass.

2. Pour in the tonic water and lemon juice and stir well.

3. Garnish with the lemon wheel.

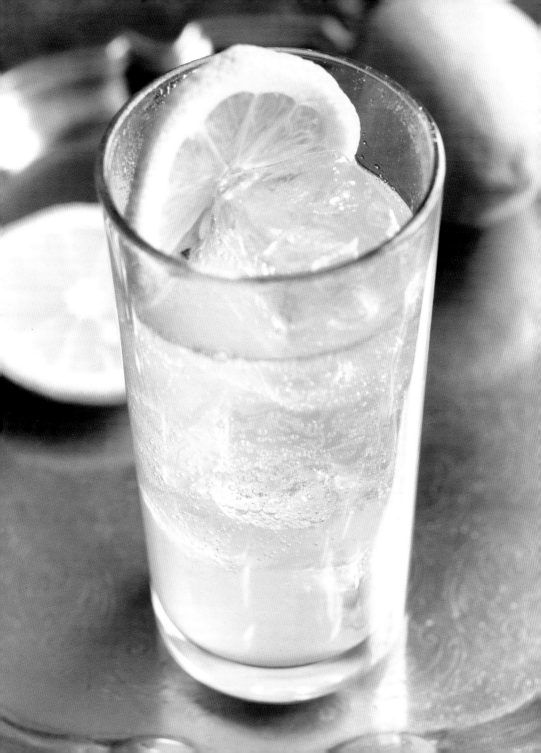

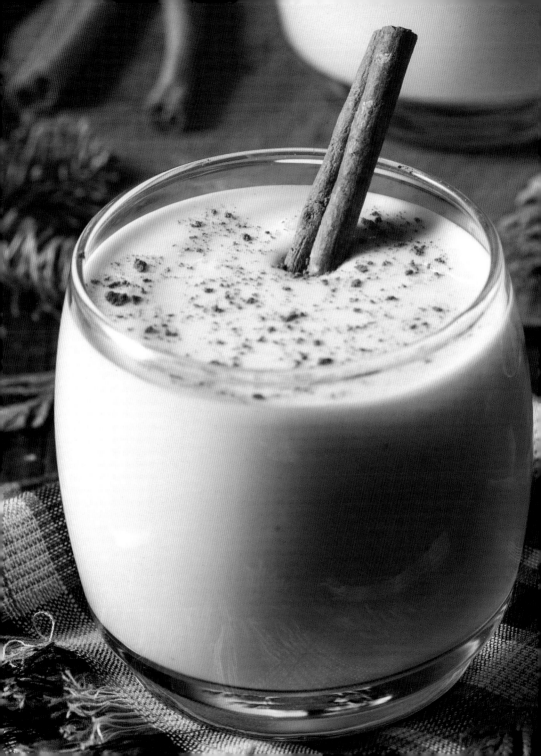

COFFEE & CINNAMON EGGNOG

Serves 4

Ingredients

2 cups milk

⅔ cup strong black coffee

1 cinnamon stick

2 extra-large eggs

⅓ cup granulated sugar

½ cup heavy cream

2 teaspoons ground cinnamon

1. Put the milk, coffee, and cinnamon stick into a saucepan and heat over medium heat until almost boiling. Cool for 5 minutes, then remove and discard the cinnamon stick.

2. Put the eggs and sugar into a bowl and beat until pale and thick. Gradually beat in the milk and coffee mixture. Return to the pan and heat gently, stirring all the time, until just thickened. Cool for 30 minutes.

3. Put the cream into a bowl and whip until it holds soft peaks. Gently fold the cream into the egg mixture. Divide among four glasses, sprinkle with ground cinnamon. Chill for 1–2 hours before serving.

DR. ESPRESSO

Serves 1

Ingredients

2 ounces espresso

1 teaspoon vanilla

6 ounces Dr. Pepper

1. In a mixing glass, stir the espresso and vanilla together with ice.

2. Fill a glass with ice and pour in the Dr. Pepper. Pour the espresso mix over the top and stir gently.

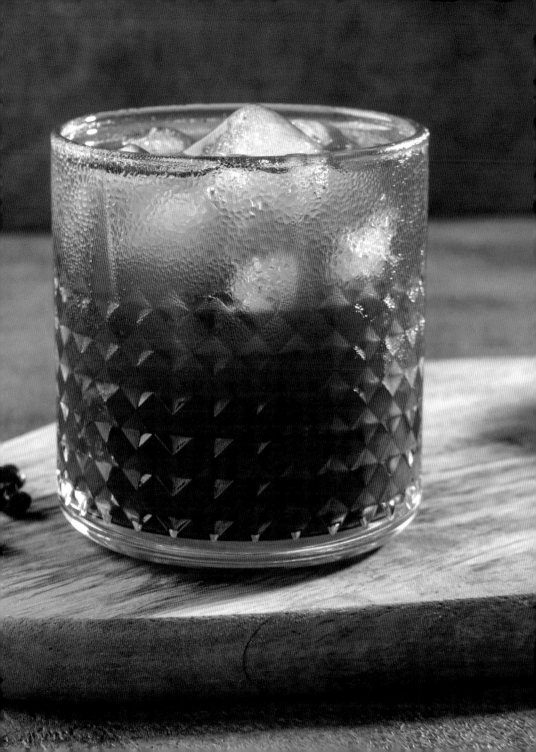

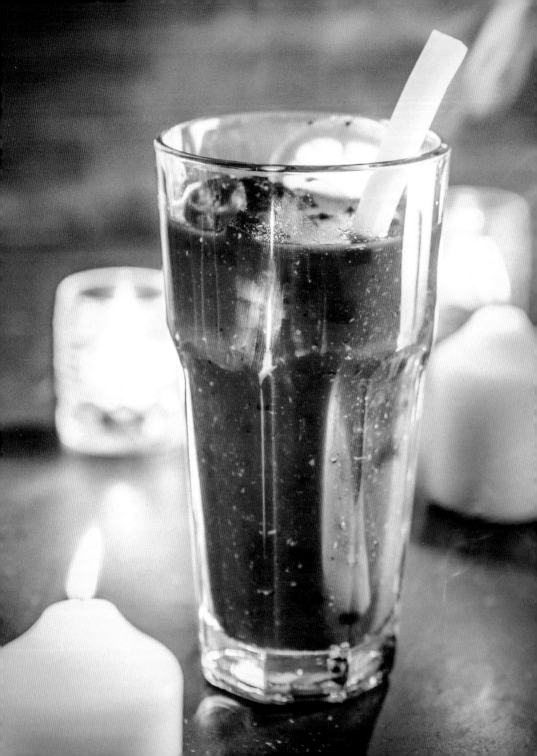

BEET VIRGIN MARY

Serves 1

Ingredients

1 ounce raw beet, peeled

6 ounces tomato juice

1 teaspoon Worcestershire sauce

¼ teaspoon celery salt

¼ teaspoon pepper

1 teaspoon horseradish, freshly grated

½ teaspoon hot pepper sauce

1 lemon slice, to garnish

celery stick, to garnish

1. Cut the beet into small pieces. Place in a cocktail shaker and crush thoroughly with a muddler or pestle to release the color and flavor.

2. Add the tomato juice, Worcestershire sauce, celery salt, pepper, horseradish, and hot pepper sauce. Stir well with a barspoon.

3. Pour the mixture into a Collins or highball glass. Add some ice cubes and stir again.

4. Garnish the drink with the lemon slice and celery stick.

CARROT CHILL

Serves 2

Ingredients

16 ounces carrot juice

1 ounce watercress

1 tablespoon lemon juice

fresh watercress
sprigs, to garnish

1. Pour the carrot juice into a blender. Add the watercress and lemon juice and process until smooth.

2. Transfer to a pitcher, cover with plastic wrap, and chill in the refrigerator for at least 1 hour.

3. Pour into glasses and garnish with watercress.

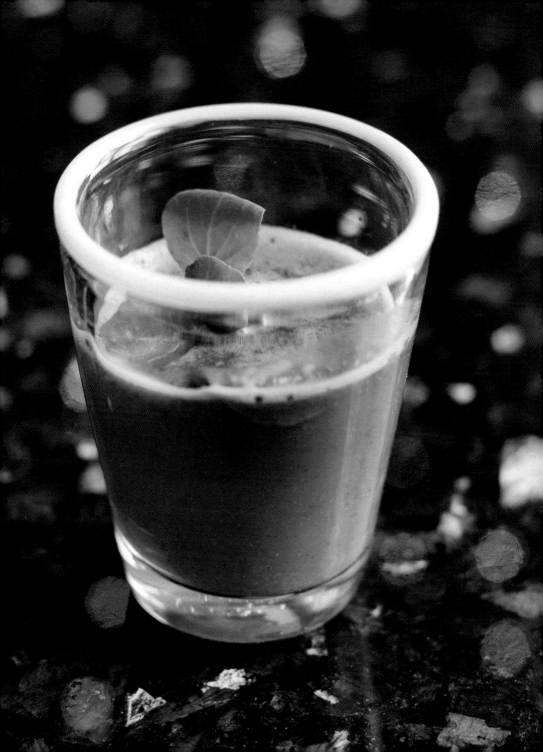

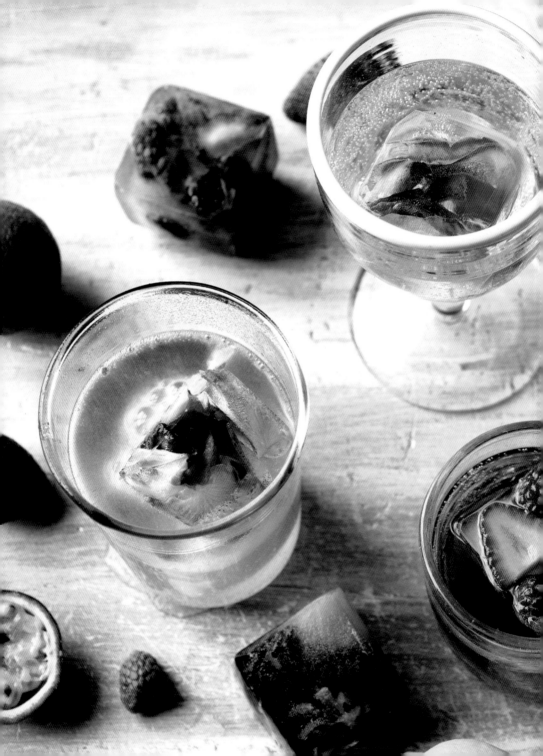

ICE
TECHNIQUES

Ice is a key ingredient in any mixed drink. Here are some of the ways that ice can be used in your mocktail. Crushed ice is generally used for frozen drinks or a julep. You can crush ice at home in a blender, although the heat from the motor can melt it quickly. Another way is to wrap cubed ice in a bag or tea towel and whack it with a mallet or rolling pin.

Flavored ice cubes can be made by filling your ice cube tray with the juice required for your mocktail. Place the filled tray in the coldest part of your freezer and leave it for at least a day—you want the cubes to be rock solid and glacially cold. These cubes mean that your mocktail will change flavor as the ice cubes melt over time.

Garnish ice is a relatively new style of ice that enhances the flavor and appearance of a mixed drink. When filling your ice cube tray, simply place a solid form into the tray before freezing. Make this something related to your mocktail, such as a berry, orange peel, rosemary, or a chili slice.

Ice balls are the latest craze in mixology and they can enhance the visual appeal of your mocktail creations. Silicone ice ball makers are widely available, but you can also use a balloon to make teardrop-shaped balls. To do this, fill round balloons with around 2 ounces of water or juice. Tie the balloons and hang them upside down in the freezer so they do not touch anything underneath. After a day or two, cut the balloon and free your frozen ice ball.

GINGER CRUSH

Serves 2

Ingredients

8 ounces carrot juice

4 tomatoes, peeled, seeded, and roughly chopped

1 tablespoon lemon juice

1 ounce fresh parsley

1 tablespoon grated fresh ginger

4 ounces water

chopped parsley, to garnish

1. Put the carrot juice, tomatoes, and lemon juice into a blender and process gently until combined.

2. Add the parsley, ginger, and 6 ice cubes. Process until well combined, pour in the water, and process until smooth.

3. Pour the mixture into tall glasses and garnish with the chopped parsley.

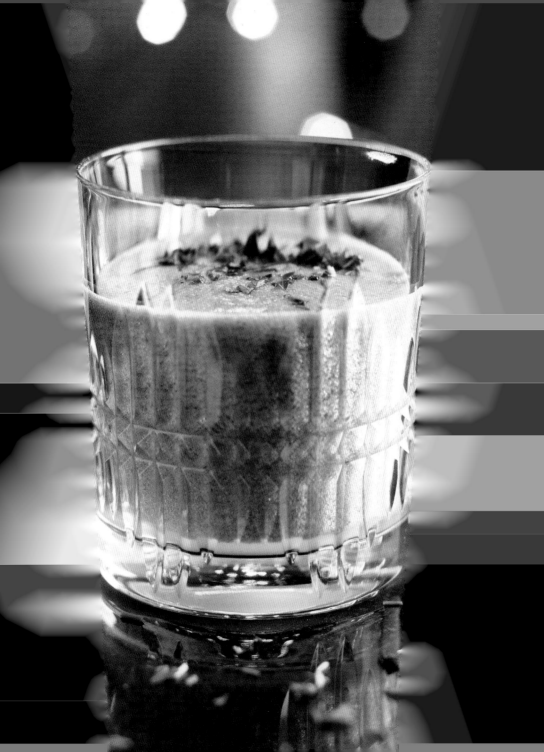

BITE OF THE APPLE

Serves 1

—

Ingredients

7½ ounces apple juice

1½ ounces lime juice

½ teaspoon orgeat syrup

1 tablespoon apple sauce
or apple puree

ground cinnamon

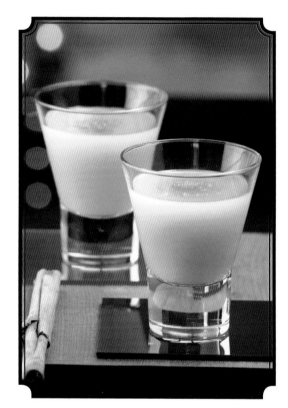

1. Blend ice in a blender with the apple juice, lime juice,
orgeat syrup, and apple sauce until smooth.

2. Pour into a chilled lowball glass and sprinkle with cinnamon.

SANGRIA SECA

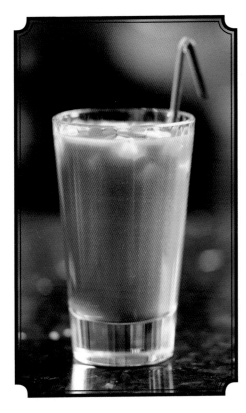

Serves 6

—

Ingredients

16 ounces tomato juice

8 ounces orange juice

4½ ounces lime juice

¾ ounce hot pepper sauce

2 teaspoons
Worcestershire sauce

1 jalapeño, deseeded
and finely chopped

celery salt and white pepper

1. Pour the tomato juice, orange juice, lime juice, hot pepper
sauce, and Worcestershire sauce into a pitcher.

2. Add the chopped jalapeño and season to taste with the celery salt and white pepper.

3. Stir well, cover, and chill in the refrigerator for at least an hour.

4. To serve, half-fill 6 highball glasses with ice and strain
the cocktail evenly into the glasses.

RANCH GIRL

Serves 1

—

Ingredients

1½ ounces lime juice

1½ ounces barbecue sauce

1 dash Worcestershire sauce

1 dash hot pepper sauce

tomato juice

lime slices, to garnish

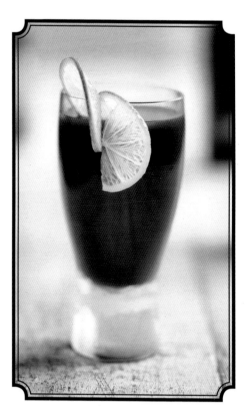

1. Shake the lime juice, barbecue sauce, Worcestershire sauce, and hot pepper sauce over ice cubes until well frosted.

2. Pour into a chilled highball glass, top with tomato juice and stir.

3. Garnish with a couple of slices of lime.

NEW ENGLAND PARTY

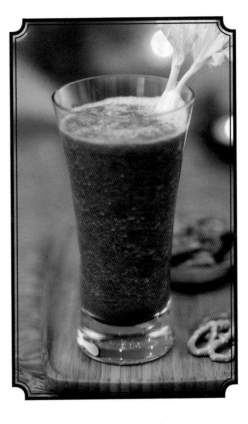

Serves 2

—

Ingredients

1 dash hot pepper sauce

1 dash Worcestershire sauce

1 teaspoon lemon juice

1 carrot, chopped

2 celery sticks, chopped

10 ounces tomato juice

5 ounces clam juice

salt and freshly ground
black pepper

celery sticks, to garnish

1. Put all the ingredients, except the seasoning and celery
stick, into a blender and blend until smooth.

2. Transfer to a jug, cover and chill in the refrigerator for about an hour.

3. Pour into two chilled highball glasses and season to taste.

4. Garnish each glass with a celery stick.

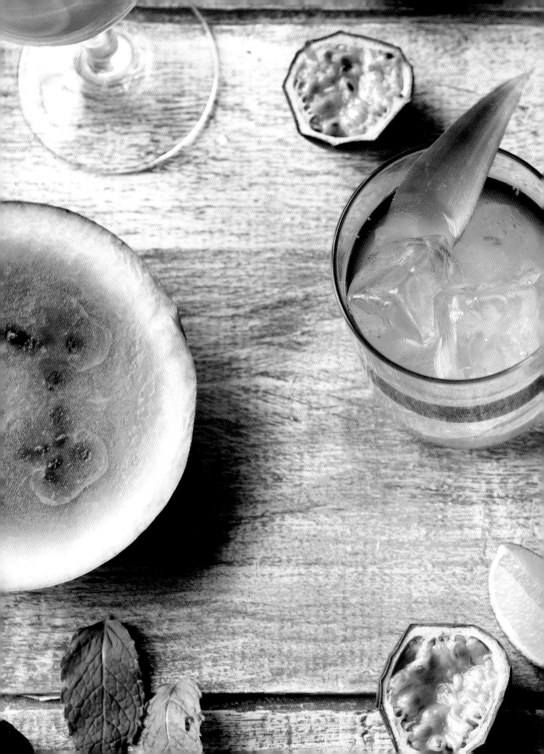

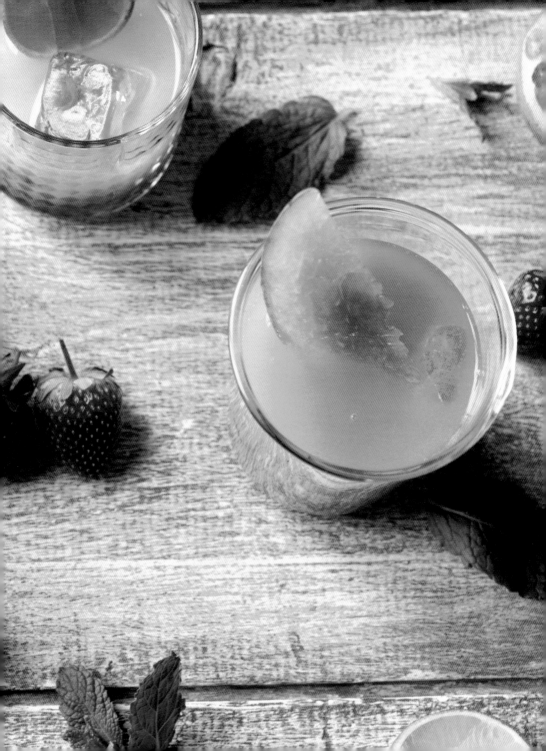

INDEX

—

This edition published by Cottage Door Press, LLC in 2024
First published 2017 by Parragon Books, Ltd.

Copyright © 2024 Cottage Door Press, LLC
5005 Newport Drive
Rolling Meadows, Illinois 60008
www.cottagedoorpress.com

Photography Mike Cooper and Günter Beer
Additional images used under license from Shutterstock.com
and istockphoto.com/Getty Images

Cover design by Bert Fanslow. Cover art used under license from Shutterstock.com

ISBN 978-1-64638-918-6

Printed in China

Art of Mixology™ is a trademark of Cottage Door Press, LLC.
Parragon Books is an imprint of Cottage Door Press, LLC.
Parragon® and the Parragon® logo are registered trademarks of Cottage Door Press, LLC.

Notes for the Reader

This book uses standard kitchen measuring spoons and cups. All spoon and cup
measurements are level unless otherwise indicated. Unless otherwise stated, milk is
assumed to be whole, eggs are large, individual vegetables are medium, and pepper
is freshly ground black pepper. Unless otherwise stated, all root vegetables should
be peeled prior to using. People with nut allergies should be aware that some of
the prepared ingredients used in the recipes in this book may contain nuts.

Recipes using raw or very lightly cooked eggs should be avoided by infants,
the elderly, pregnant women, and people with weakened immune systems.

Garnishes, decorations, and serving suggestions are all optional and not necessarily
included in the recipe ingredients or method. The times given are only an approximate
guide. Preparation times differ according to the techniques used by different people
and the cooking times may also vary from those given. Optional ingredients,
variations, or serving suggestions have not been included in the time calculations.

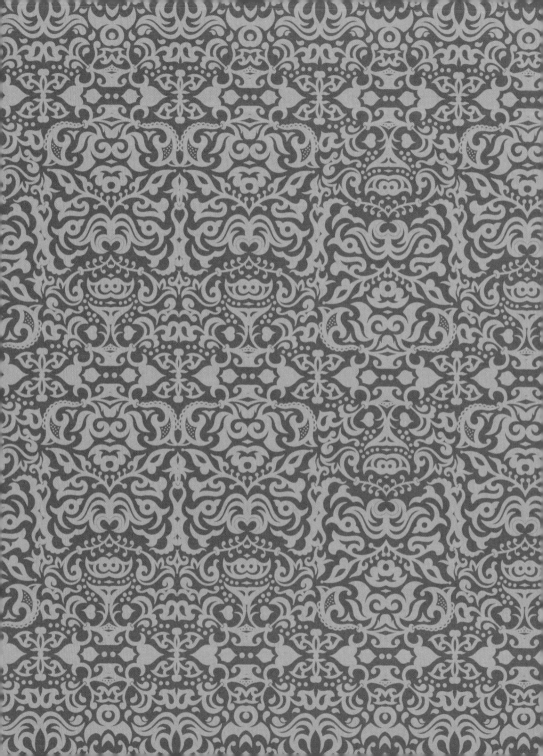